Step by Step®

Management of Cubitus Varus by Ilizarov Technique

Step by Step®
Management of Cubitus Varus by Ilizarov Technique

RA Agrawal
MS(Orthopaedics) AO/ASIF(Germany, Austria) Ilizarov(Russia)
Director
Agrawal Orthopedic Hospital
Gorakhpur, Uttar Pradesh, India
Past President, ASAMI India

Sureshwar Pandey
MS(Surgery, Orthopedic) FICS FIAMS FAC FAS FACS FNAMS
Ex-Head and Emeritus Professor
Department of Orthopedics
Rajendra Medical College and Hospital
Ranchi, Jharkhand, India
Emeritus President, Indian Foot and Ankle Society

Rajat Agrawal
MS(Orthopedics)
Senior Orthopedic Surgeon
Agrawal Orthopedic Hospital
Gorakhpur, Uttar Pradesh, India
President, ASAMI India (2023–2025)

JAYPEE

JAYPEE BROTHERS MEDICAL PUBLISHERS
The Health Sciences Publisher
New Delhi | London

Jaypee Brothers Medical Publishers (P) Ltd

Headquarters

EMCA House
23/23-B, Ansari Road, Daryaganj
New Delhi 110 002, India
Landline: +91-11-23272143, +91-11-23272703
+91-11-23282021, +91-11-23245672
E-mail: jaypee@jaypeebrothers.com

Corporate Office

Jaypee Brothers Medical Publishers (P) Ltd.
4838/24, Ansari Road, Daryaganj
New Delhi 110 002, India
Phone: +91-11-43574357
Fax: +91-11-43574314
E-mail: jaypee@jaypeebrothers.com

Overseas Office

JP Medical Ltd.
83, Victoria Street, London
SW1H 0HW (UK)
Phone: +44-20 3170 8910
Fax: +44(0)20 3008 6180
E-mail: info@jpmedpub.com

Website: www.jaypeebrothers.com

Website: www.jaypeedigital.com

Inquiries for bulk sales may be solicited at: jaypee@jaypeebrothers.com

***Step by Step® Management of Cubitus Varus by Ilizarov Technique* / RA Agrawal, Sureshwar Pandey, Rajat Agrawal**

First Edition: **2025**

ISBN: 978-93-6616-226-3

Printed at: Samrat Offset Pvt. Ltd.

Preface

A deformity in whatever form, at whichever site, and in whatever age is not acceptable by anyone. Not surprisingly, in the precivilization era, the disabled persons were put to crucible tests for survivorship; that is, if they could work hard, earn their livelihood, and help their community in their needs, then only they had the right to survive. On the other hand, those who could not prove their worth on the above fronts were done to death. Deformities produce physical disfigurement and physical disabilities. They also produce psychological depression, need more energy consumption in executing even the routine functions, and subsequently lead to secondary deformities locally and even distantly resulting into ultimate premature degenerative changes in various joints. Therefore, any deformity must be corrected as far as possible. With the dawn of the civilization, the disabled persons started to expect their right to survive in the world. Gradually, the society started to accept them, treat them, rehabilitate them, and provide them the dignity of life. Ultimately, the medical world took the challenge of preventing, managing, and rehabilitating these disabled/deformed persons. There has been variable success on all fronts. However, the maximum success has been achieved in correcting and minimizing the deformity. In this very direction, the birth of the "third dimension (rehabilitation medicine) of medicine" took place. Most of the initial deformities are amenable to controlled, graduated, stretching schedule and proper physiotherapy. However, as the deformities advance, they become stiff and some semi-invasive or invasive method for management has to be employed.

The old standard treatment method includes corrective osteotomy followed by plaster fixation. Gradually, the stabilization of the osteotomy is setting implants like K-wires, screws, wires, and plate fixation. The first description of lateral closed wedge osteotomy for cubitus varus was reported by Siris in 1939. Since then, various procedures of osteotomy were described, but complication rates were about 30% because osteotomy was performed in very thin bone. All the osteotomies were performed by open surgeries. Ilizarov has mentioned percutaneous osteotomy with distraction osteogenesis. This helps a lot in bringing the normal architecture of the bone.

In this very direction, the Kurgan surgeon GA Ilizarov introduced his technique for tackling various problems and one of them has been for the correction of fixed deformity. The principle behind the Ilizarov technique has great depth. However, against the speed with which the Ilizarov technique was accepted all over the world, its decline unfortunately is also being palpably observed. There can be several reasons but its overuse, uncalculated use, misuse, and underuse have a definite role to play for its decline. And nonetheless, the improper passing of K-wire, injudicious selection of point of entry of wires, and improper placement of rings have a definite role to play in bringing disrepute to the Ilizarov technique. Let us not blame the young enthusiastic surgeons who want to master any technology in minimum time and effort. We feel that there is hardly any monograph detailing the basics of the Ilizarov technique, which includes acquaintance with the hardware, proper selection of patient, pinpointing the placement of the K-wires and the direction of the wire advancement. Another disadvantage is the steep learning curve, so that in most situations successful management of complex deformities can be achieved only after years of experience.

The biomechanics itself is a tough subject and we want to avoid intricacies of the biomechanics in our practical life. However, the understanding of the basic kinematics, anatomical localization of the suitable points, and basic physiology of execution of function are mandatory before attempting to master any technique.

We have tried to tackle the above problems in a lucid and descriptive manner, so that this manual may be useful even to the beginners, who want to know, learn, execute, and get effective result after the use of the Ilizarov technique.

We all want to put our best to make this monograph acceptable by all; however, there may be many shortcomings for which apology is solicited. In preparing this monograph, we have consulted many books and journals, derived in ideas and inspiration, and have been educated through different sources. However, we are particularly indebted to the books given in bibliography, which we have consulted several times. We have no hesitation in giving full credit to these sources.

We are highly thankful to young and enthusiastic orthopaedic surgeon **Dr Raju Bollabathini (MS Ortho) and Dr Ashish Agrahari (MS Ortho)** whose dedication and hard work has made the writing of this book possible.

We acknowledge the constant help of our sincere colleagues and friends like VK Shahi (PT), Mr Anoop, Mr Abhay Mishra, and Mr Santosh (artist).

The typing, aligning the manuscript, and improving the script comprise the real tough job in preparing any book, and all that have been done tirelessly by Ms Smita Dubey and Huma Fatima (PT) who remained alert and active for this work at all the time.

The authors could not have concentrated on the work unless the family members had provided them full cooperation. And to this, the dear family of Dr RA Agrawal has stood the test of time accepting all the eccentricities during the preparation of this book. The contribution of Dr RA Agrawal's wife Mrs Rashmi, son Dr Rajat, the young budding orthopedic surgeon, and daughter Mrs Richa, the software engineer, simply deserve all credit in uninterrupted production of this book.

RA Agrawal
Sureshwar Pandey
Rajat Agrawal

Contents

CHAPTER

1 Introduction

Cubitus varus is the most common angular deformity that results from supracondylar fractures in children. This is usually late sequelae for poorly treated or those in which reduction was lost without observation. There may be other reasons for this deformity, however, most understood reason is malunited medially displaced and medially rotated distal fragment. Smith (1960) proved in his experimental studies that varus tilting of the distal fragment was the most important cause of the change in the carrying angle and showed that rotation of distal fragment was most important condition leading to this deformity. Le belle et al. found varus tilting of the distal fragment in all their patients, with cubitus varus after supracondylar fractures. Several types of treatment have been described for cubitus varus deformity such as lateral closed wedge osteotomy, dome osteotomy, complex multiplanar osteotomy, distraction osteogenesis, and opening medial wedge osteotomy. However, method preferred by most surgeons is lateral closing wedge osteotomy. The method of fixation ranged from plate and screw fixation, Kirschner wire fixation, external fixation that ranging from simple uniplanar fixator to Ilizarov ring fixators. However, complications associated in these fixations vary from under- or overcorrection, failure of fixation, neuropraxia, an unsightly scar, refracture at the osteotomy site, limitation of range of movement at the elbow, infection, etc. All these treatment modalities achieve definitive correction to a variable extent in single stage and for the residuals another definitive surgery has to be done. Ilizarov technique corrects the residual deformities by offering three-dimensional corrections. However, any further surgical correction should be undertaken only after maximum auto remodeling, which may take round about a year. For any further surgery or revision surgery, patients demand growth potential and status of physis must be considered.

WHEN TO DO THE SURGERY?

Surgery should be done only after allowing for maximum remodeling. A rough estimate will be around a year after the original injury. Again, patients demand, growth potential, and status of physis should be taken into account while planning for surgery.

WHAT SURGERIES ARE AVAILABLE?

Surgeries available for correction of cubitus varus are medial opening wedge osteotomy (King and Secor, 1951), the lateral closing wedge osteotomy (French, 1959), the oblique osteotomy of Amspacher and Messenbaugh (1964), the step cut osteotomy (De Rosa and Grazanio, 1988), the dome osteotomy (Kanaujia, 1988), the pentalateral osteotomy (Laupattarakasem, 1989), and the three-dimensional osteotomy (Uchida, 1991). However, the preferred method being practiced by many is the lateral wedge closing osteotomy. However, several authors have reported poor cosmetic appearance due to lateral condylar prominence. Despite being an effective means of correction of the varus deformity, several authors have reported a poor cosmetic appearance due to lateral condylar prominence. Furthermore, the tendency of the distal fragment to angulate into varus following internal fixation by screws or staples often leads to varus angulation of the distal fragment. To avoid this complication, external fixation devices (like simple uniplanar fixator to circular fixator) may be used as an alternative method of fixation to avoid recurrence of the deformity. This has led to the emergence of external fixation, which may range from simple uniplanar fixators to circular fixators, as an alternative modality of fixation of the osteotomy. Among the many external fixations, Ilizarov circular fixator has advantage of correcting the deformity in three planes. Unlike single stage surgical procedure, which is achieved as an acute correction of the deformity and impedes any further corrections, the method of compression-distraction osteogenesis using external fixation is the only treatment modality enabling further adjustments to be made postoperatively. Postsurgical frame modifications are easily performed, as desired, in the outpatient department. However, this method is associated with its own share of complications such as over- or undercorrection, failure of fixation, unsightly scars, refractures, functional restriction of movements, and infections.

CLOSED WEDGE SUPRACONDYLAR OSTEOTOMY

- The supracondylar fracture is usually at the olecranon fossa, thus center of rotation of axis (CORA) is in the olecranon fossa. In the closed wedge osteotomy, wedge-shaped bone piece is removed in supracondylar region. The principle of osteotomy is—if the osteotomy is

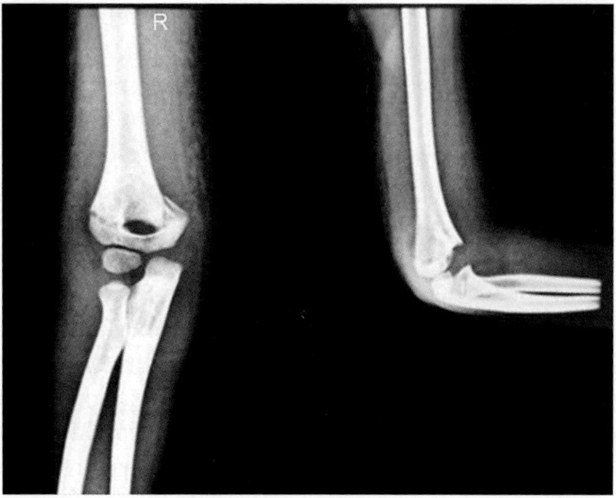

Fig. 1.1: Malunited supracondylar humerus.

performed at the CORA, there will be no translation of fragment **(Fig. 1.1)**.

- Osteotomy is performed above the CORA, according to the principle of osteotomy rule 2, there should be medial translation of the lower fragment while correcting the varus deformity.
- In closed wedge osteotomy, which is performed at the supracondylar region, there is no provision of the translation of the lower fragment.
- In closed wedge osteotomy, the width of the lower fragment is larger than the proximal fragment which leads to prominence of lateral condyle.
- Since medial translation of the lower fragment is not done, it leads to "lazy S" deformity.

- Osteotomy is performed in a very thin bone, thus, there is difficulty to reduce the fragment and maintain the stability of the fragment.
- Since the fracture is not stable at osteotomy site, there is chance of recurrence of the deformity.
- The varus deformity is corrected acutely, so undercorrection and overcorrection cannot be managed.
- The distal fragment is unstable, there is more chance of the nonunion.

DEFORMITY CORRECTED BY MONOLATERAL FIXATOR

- In monolateral fixator, deformity can be corrected acutely or gradually, but there is no provision of the medial translation which does not follow the principle of osteotomy rule 2.
- There is no provision for correction of the internal rotation deformity.
- The fixator is monolateral, thus the fixator is mechanically unstable.

ILIZAROV DISTRACTION OSTEOGENESIS

Distraction osteogenesis has several advantages in deformity surgery such as providing adjustable, three-dimensional correction, stable fixation, and allowing immediate range of motion (ROM) with less soft tissue damage and scar formation. Distraction osteogenesis is a slow process but very stable. There are less chances of displacement of the fragment. As the incision is very small, periosteum is not very much disturbed. Good amount of callus is usually formed. There are less chances of the nerve injury, secondly there is gradual distraction of the soft tissues so the blood vessels and nerves are gradually distracted. There are less chances of neuropraxia. The blood vascularity is increased due to gradual distraction. The Ilizarov frame is quite stable. The physiotherapy is started when the pain subsides. The distraction osteogenesis produces the good callus formation. Postoperative complications such as stiffness of the joints, numbness, and tingling of limb are not found. If numbness and tingling occur immediately, distraction is stopped. The distraction is started after 2–3 days, when the things become normal, again physiotherapy is started.

CHAPTER

2 Anatomy of Elbow Joint

INTRODUCTION

The elbow is a complex hinge joint composed of humero-ulnar, humeroradial, and proximal radioulnar articulations which share a common synovial cavity. Humeroulnar and humeroradial are the principal articulations and allow flexion and extension at elbow, whereas proximal radioulnar joint is involved with pronation and supination of forearm. The joint line is situated 2 cm below the line joining the two epicondyles and slopes downward and medially.

OSSIFICATION

The elbow develops from multiple secondary ossification centers appearing at different ages and fusing together around maturity. A knowledge of normal epiphysis and apophysis, age of their appearance, and their relationship to the bone is of utmost importance for correct interpretation of a radiograph of pediatric elbow. The approximate ages of appearance of the secondary ossification **(Fig. 2.1)** centers around the elbow joint are:

- Capitulum—1 year
- Radial head—3 years
- Internal (medial) epicondyle—5 years
- Trochlea—7 years

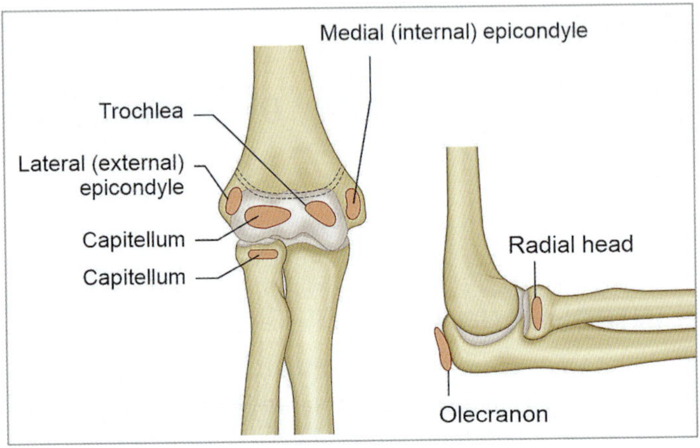

Fig. 2.1: Ossification of elbow.

- Olecranon—9 years
- External (lateral) epicondyle—11 years

This sequence of appearance can be remembered by mnemonic CRITOE. They may appear at a younger age in girls (6–12 months ahead of their male counterpart). However, the sequence remains constant.

OSTEOLOGY

Humeroulnar Joint

The humeroulnar joint is a uniaxial, diarthrodial joint between trochlea of distal humerus and trochlear notch of proximal ulna allowing flexion and extension. Although generally described as a hinge joint, it is probably more appropriately designated as a modified hinge joint, with small amounts (approximately 5°) of internal and external rotation occurring at the extremes of flexion and extension. The trochlea is hourglass shaped with a central depression called the trochlear groove bound on either side by two unequal, convex segments of bone. This groove is obliquely arranged, running from anterior to posterior, an obliquity which has individual variation and may account for variations in the carrying angle.

Immediately above the articular surfaces of the humerus, on the anterior side, is a bony depression called coronoid fossa which receives coronoid process of the ulna during flexion. Posteriorly, the olecranon fossa receives the olecranon process of the ulna during extension. The proximal ulna has a central trochlear ridge that runs between the olecranon posteriorly and the coronoid process anteriorly. On either side of this ridge is a concave region known as the trochlear notch, which corresponds to the convex surface of the humeral trochlea. The structural congruency of these articular surfaces makes the humeroulnar joint one of the most stable joints in the human musculoskeletal system.

Another significant anatomical feature is the medial epicondyle, a bony prominence located proximal and medial to the trochlea. The medial epicondyle serves as the attachment point for flexor-pronator muscle group and ulnar collateral ligament. This prominence continues superiorly to form the medial supracondylar ridge. Just posterior to the medial epicondyle is the cubital tunnel or ulna groove, a bony depression that protects and houses the ulnar nerve **(Figs. 2.2 to 2.5)**.

Humeroradial Joint

The humeroradial joint, like the humeroulnar joint, is a diarthrodial uniaxial joint. However, it performs a dual role

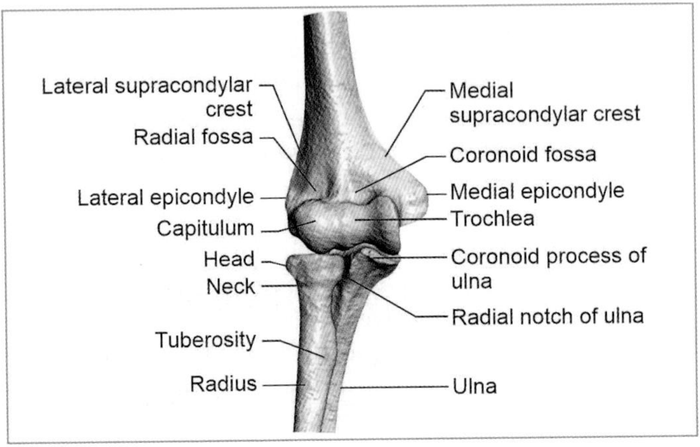

Fig. 2.2: Anterior view.

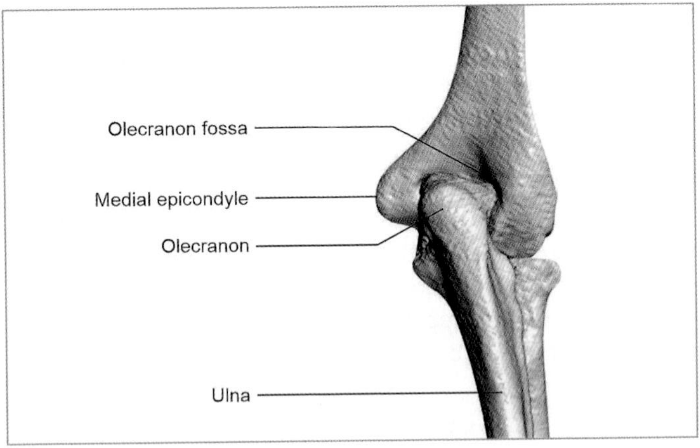

Fig. 2.3: Posterior view.

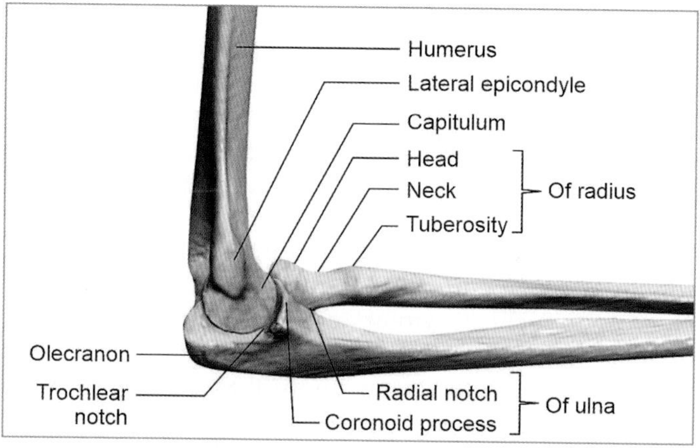

Fig. 2.4: Medial view.

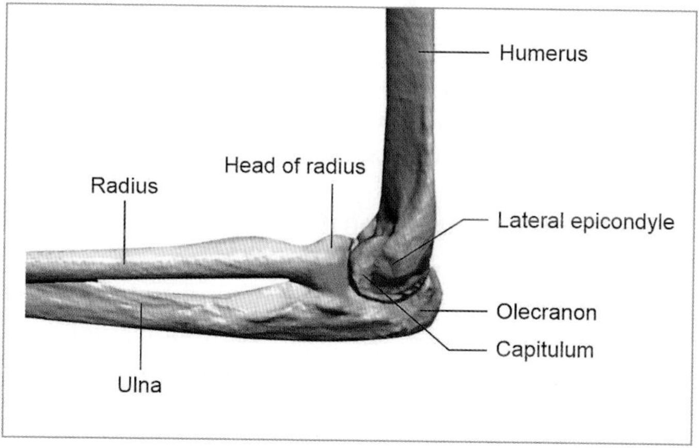

Fig. 2.5: Osteology of Elbow. Lateral view.

in that it glides around a coronal axis to perform flexion/extension movements with the humeroulnar joint and pivots around a longitudinal axis to perform rotational movements in association with the superior radioulnar joint. Thus, this joint is often referred to as a hinge/pivot joint. The articular structures include capitulum of distal humerus and upper surface of radial head. The capitulum is not a complete sphere but, actually, an anterior half of a sphere. Unlike the trochlea, it does not extend posteriorly. The capitotrochlear groove separating capitulum from trochlea guides the rim of radial head as it moves in flexion and extension. Immediately above the capitulum on the anterior aspect of the humerus is a depression called the radial fossa. This fossa receives the anterior tip of the radial head in the fully flexed position. Lateral to the radial fossa is a bony prominence known as the lateral epicondyle which serves as point of attachment for common extensor group of muscles. This prominence extends superiorly as the lateral supracondylar ridge. The radial head and its surrounding rim narrow distally to form the radial neck. The radial head and neck are not collinear but form an angle of 15° with respect to the shaft of radius.

Superior Radioulnar Joint

The superior radioulnar joint functions with inferior radioulnar joint to produce rotation of forearm (supination and pronation). This uniaxial, diarthrodial joint is comprised of the convex medial rim of the radial head and the concave radial notch of the ulna. During rotation, the radius crosses over the ulna and the head of the radius rotates within a ring formed by the annular ligament (AL) and radial notch of the ulna.

Carrying Angle

The carrying angle of elbow is the angle between long axis of arm and forearm resulting in an abducted position of forearm relative to arm. It is measured in frontal plane with elbow extended and forearm fully supinated. The medial flange of trochlea is 6 mm deeper than its lateral flange. Furthermore, superior articular surface of coronoid process is placed obliquely in relation to long axis of ulna. These two factors together are responsible for a carrying angle. Its value ranges between 5 and 15° and is slightly greater in female than in male and greater on nondominant side than in dominant arm **(Fig. 2.6)**.

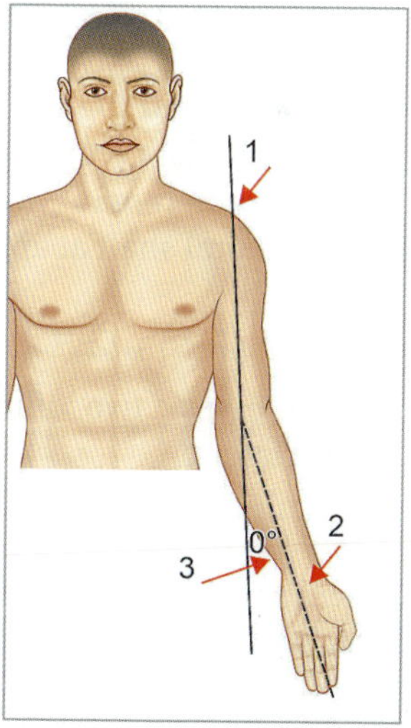

Fig. 2.6: Carrying angle; 1—long axis of arm, 2—long axis of forearm, 3—carrying angle.

Tri-column Concept of Distal Humerus

Anatomically, the distal humerus is triangular in shape consisting of two columns and a "tie arch". The medial column holds at its distal end the medial epicondyle and medial part of trochlea. The lateral column at its distal end has capitulum and lateral epicondyle more proximally. The articular segment functions architecturally as a tie arch. This arrangement is crucial for stable elbow movement and should be restored in case of distal humerus fracture **(Figs. 2.7A and B)**.

From a lateral perspective, the articular surface of the trochlea and capitulum is projected anteriorly at an angle of 40° to the axis of the humerus, the trochlear axis being externally rotated at an angle of 3–8° and compared with the longitudinal axis being in 4–8° of valgus. The medial epicondyle lies on the projected axis of the shaft, whereas the lateral epicondyle is projected slightly forward from the axis. In frontal plane, the medial column diverges from the humeral shaft at approximately 45°, whereas the lateral column diverges from humeral shaft at approximately 20°.

Ligamentous Support (Figs. 2.8 and 2.9)

The elbow joint possesses two main ligamentous complexes—medial and lateral.

Medial Side

On the medial side, *ulnar collateral ligament (UCL)* consists of three parts—anterior oblique, posterior oblique, and transverse portion.

- *Anterior oblique bundle* is the deepest layer and most important support on medial side. It originates from the inferior surface of medial epicondyle and inserts on the

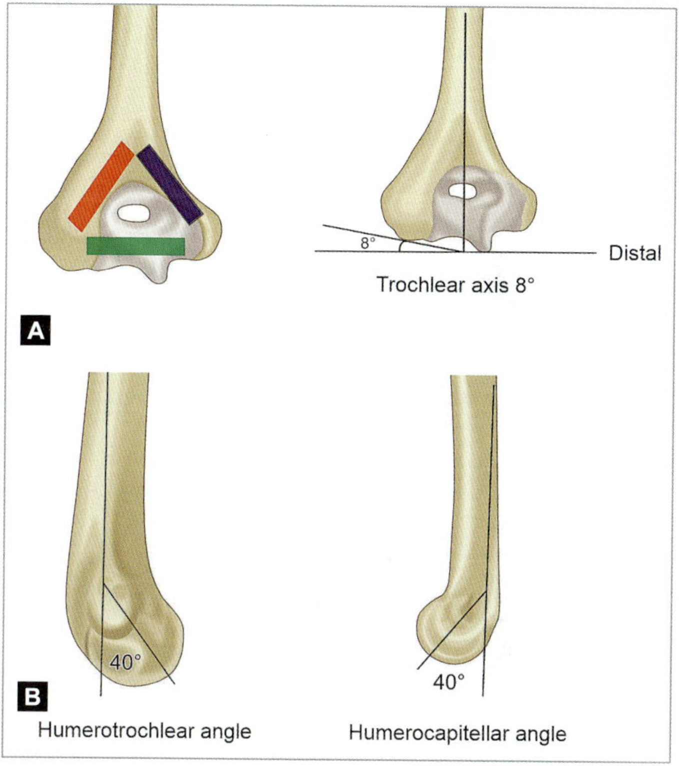

Figs. 2.7A and B: Anatomy of distal humerus. (A) Tri-column of distal humerus and (B) Condylar arrangement.

medial aspect of coronoid process. The humeral origin is located just posterior in relation to the axis of rotation and this eccentric position permits tautness to the ligament throughout the range of motion. Its compromise leads to gross valgus instability in all positions of elbow except extension.

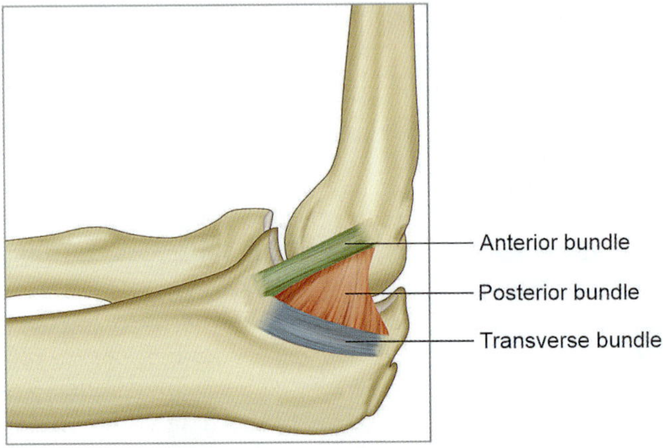

Fig. 2.8: Ulnar collateral ligament of elbow.

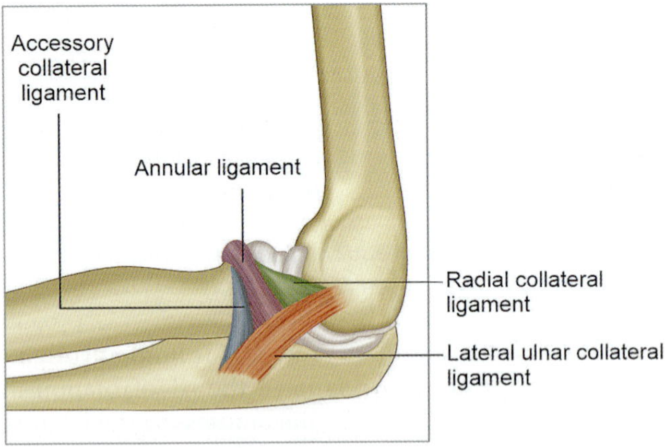

Fig. 2.9: Lateral ligamentous complex of elbow.

- *The posterior oblique bundle* is fan-shaped structure and originates from medial epicondyle, posterior and inferior to the axis of rotation and further distant from its anterior oblique counterpart. It inserts into the posteromedial aspect of olecranon. The more eccentric location of origin in relation to axis of rotation provides it greater variance in length. This portion of UCL becomes taut in flexion. However, its compromise does not affect the medial stability significantly.
- *The transverse bundle* of UCL originates from medial olecranon and inserts into the coronoid process of ulna. This often cannot be separated from the medial joint capsule and contributes very little to elbow stability.

Lateral Side

The lateral ligament complex is more variable than its medial counterpart and usually has four components. They are radial collateral ligament (RCL), lateral ulnar collateral ligament (LUCL), accessory lateral collateral ligament (ALCL), and AL.

- *The radial collateral ligament* originates from the lateral epicondyle directly at the axis of rotation, fans distally and inserts into the AL. It maintains close apposition of articular surfaces and provides varus stability to the humeroradial articulation of elbow.
- *The lateral ulnar collateral ligament* originates from the middle of lateral epicondyle and inserts into the tubercle of crista musculi supinatoris on ulna. Release of this structure leads to an inferior rotatory instability of humeroulnar joint. This type of subluxation is known as the *pivot shift phenomenon of elbow* and occurs even in the presence of an intact RCL.

- *The accessory lateral collateral ligament* originates from the inferior margin of AL and inserts into the tubercle of supinator crest on ulna. It becomes taut on varus stress and is not affected by movement of elbow. Functionally, it augments the AL during varus stress.
- *Annular ligament* encircles and stabilizes the radial head in the radial notch of ulna. It originates from anterior margin of radial notch and inserts on the posterior margin of radial notch making about four-fifths of a circle. The anterior and posterior portions of AL become taut in extreme supination and pronation, respectively. Other ligaments that stabilize the superior radioulnar joint are quadrate ligament and oblique cord but their functional contribution is believed to be minimal.

Neurovascular Structures Around Elbow

The elbow joint has four important nerves in its proximity. They are—median, radial, musculocutaneous, and ulnar nerve.

Median Nerve (C5, C6, C7, C8, and T1)

The median nerve lies on the anteromedial aspect of cubital fossa, medial to the biceps tendon and brachial artery. From the antecubital fossa, it continues under the bicipital aponeurosis and passes between the two heads of pronator teres. Just inferior to the border of the pronator teres, the anterior interosseous branch arises and descends along the anterior aspect of the interosseous membrane. The median nerve can be compressed between the two heads of the pronator teres or the lacertus fibrosus (bicipital aponeurosis). Compression at these points results in either the pronator syndrome or anterior interosseous syndrome. In approximately 1% of the population, an anomalous structure called the ligament of Struthers is present which can cause neurological compression of the median nerve known as supracondylar process syndrome.

Ulnar Nerve (C8 and T1)

Ulnar nerve enters the posterior compartment of arm through arcade of Struthers located 8 cm proximal to medial epicondyle. At the elbow, it is located on posteromedial aspect behind the medial epicondyle and continues down through the cubital tunnel. The nerve then enters forearm by passing between two heads of flexor carpi ulnaris muscle. Cubital tunnel is the most frequent site for ulnar nerve injury by compression or stretching. Volume of this tunnel is significantly reduced during flexion and abduction activities of elbow like throwing. Degenerative and reactive changes in nearby bone can also cause ulnar nerve irritation. Compression neuritis can also occur at arcade of Struthers or between the two heads of flexor carpi ulnaris.

Radial Nerve (C5, C6, C7, C8, and T1)

Radial nerve enters anterior compartment after piercing lateral intermuscular septum 5 cm below deltoid tuberosity. At elbow, it lies in cubital fossa between brachialis and brachioradialis, anterior to lateral epicondyle of humerus. At the level of radiocapitellar joint, it divides into posterior interosseous and superficial radial branches. The superficial radial nerve continues distally running under brachioradialis and over supinator and pronator teres muscles. The posterior interosseous branch curves around the posterior and lateral aspect of radial neck and passes between two heads of supinator muscle. It continues distally and emerges in the dorsal compartment of forearm approximately 8 cm below the elbow joint and divides into terminal motor branches. In around 50% of individuals, superior edge of supinator forms a fibrous band (arcade of Frohse/supinator arch). This is a common site for entrapment of posterior interosseous nerve.

Musculocutaneous Nerve (C5, C6, and C7)

It runs in the anterior compartment of arm between biceps and brachialis muscle to reach on the lateral side of biceps tendon. It then pierces the brachial fascia 2 cm above elbow joint and continues as the lateral cutaneous nerve of forearm. Musculocutaneous nerve can be entrapped between biceps and brachialis fascia particularly in a position of hyperextension and pronation.

Brachial Artery

Brachial artery is located on the anterior aspect of elbow medial to the tendon of biceps brachii. It is superficial throughout its extent and can be palpated in front of elbow. At the level of neck of radius, it ends by dividing into two terminal branches, the radial and ulnar arteries.

Anastomosis around Elbow Joint

Anastomosis around elbow joint links the brachial artery with the upper ends of radial and ulnar arteries. It can be divided into those situated in front and those behind the medial and lateral epicondyles of humerus. It supplies the ligaments and bones of elbow joint **(Fig. 2.10)**.

Relations of Elbow Joint

- *Anterior*: Brachialis, biceps tendon, brachial artery, and median nerve
- *Posterior*: Triceps and anconeus
- *Medially*: Common flexors and ulnar nerve

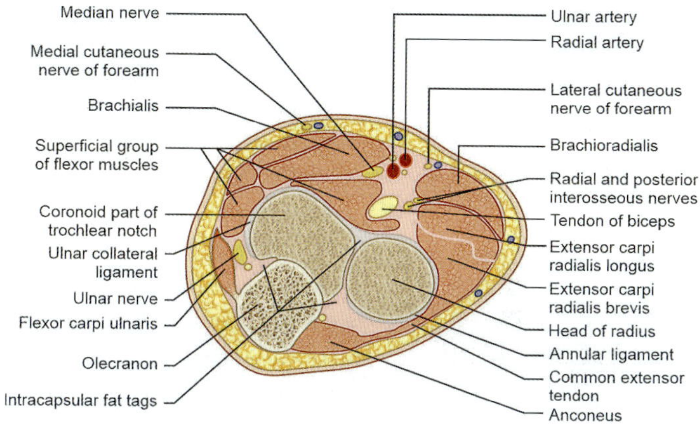

Fig. 2.10: Transverse section of the left elbow joint view from above to show the relation of the joint.

- *Laterally*: Common extensors, supinator, and radial nerve with its superficial and deep branches

Movements

Details of movements occurring at elbow joint are given in **Table 2.1**. Pronation and supination do not occur at elbow joint. They happen at proximal and distal radioulnar joints.

Bursae (Fig. 2.11)

Elbow joint is surrounded by many bursae. They protect elbow by acting as a cushion, decrease friction, and thereby limit degenerative changes. They can become inflamed and painful leading to bursitis. Elbow bursae which are of clinical importance are:

- *Intratendinous olecranon bursa*—located within the tendon of the triceps brachii near its insertion onto the olecranon

TABLE 2.1: Movements at elbow joint.

Movements	Normal range	Muscles and their nerve supply
Flexion	0–145°	• Biceps brachii (MC) • Brachialis (MC, R) • Brachioradialis (R)
Extension	145–0°	• Triceps brachii (R) • Anconeus (R)
Pronation	0–80°	• Pronator quadratus (AI) • Pronator teres (M)
Supination	0–80°	• Supinator (PI) • Biceps brachii (MC)

(MC: musculocutaneous; R: radial; AI: anterior interosseous; M: median; PI: posterior interosseous)

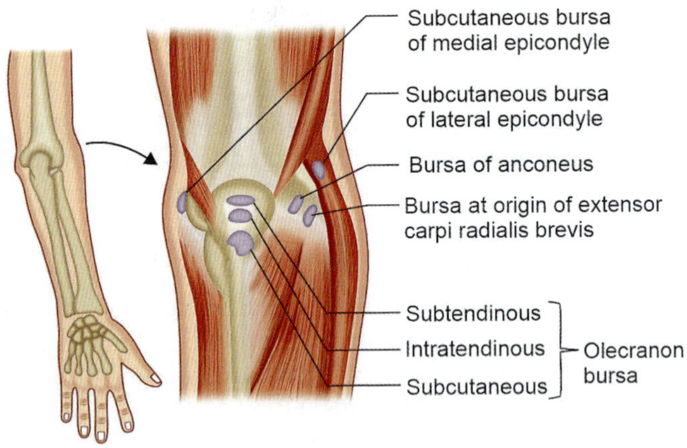

Fig. 2.11: Bursae around elbow joint.

- *Subtendinous olecranon bursa*—between the olecranon and the tendon of the triceps brachii, reducing friction between the two structures during extension and flexion of the arm.
- *Subcutaneous olecranon bursa*: It is located at the bony tip of elbow between olecranon process and the overlying connective tissue.
- *Bicipitoradial bursa*—located between distal biceps tendon and radial tuberosity. It ensures frictionless motion between the biceps tendon and the proximal radius during pronation and supination of the forearm.

Radiographic Pearls

Standard radiographic evaluation of elbow includes an anteroposterior (AP) and a lateral view image **(Fig. 2.12)**.

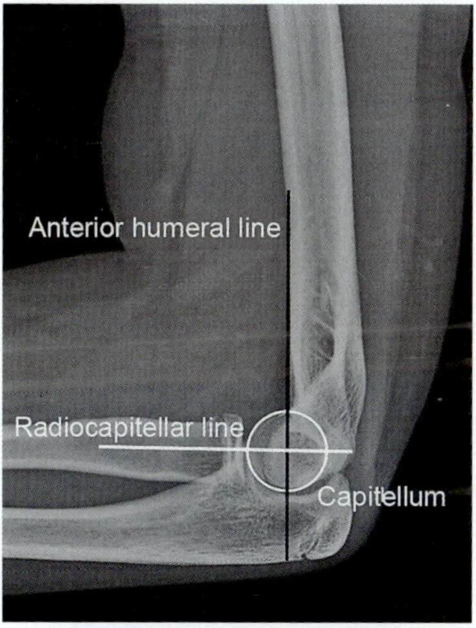

Fig. 2.12: Anterior humeral line and radiocapitellar line.

Alignment

Alignment of elbow can be evaluated on a radiograph by following parameters:

- *Anterior humeral line*: A line drawn along the anterior cortex of humerus on a lateral view should intersect the middle third of capitulum.
- *Radiocapitellar line*: A line drawn along the long axis of radius in any view passes through the middle of capitulum.
- *Humerus-elbow-wrist (HEW) angle*: It is the angle between longitudinal axis of humeral shaft and a line passing through the midpoints of two transverse lines across the forearm. It is measured on an AP view with elbow in full extension and full supination. The average value for HEW angle is 12° valgus (range 5–20°) **(Fig. 2.13)**.

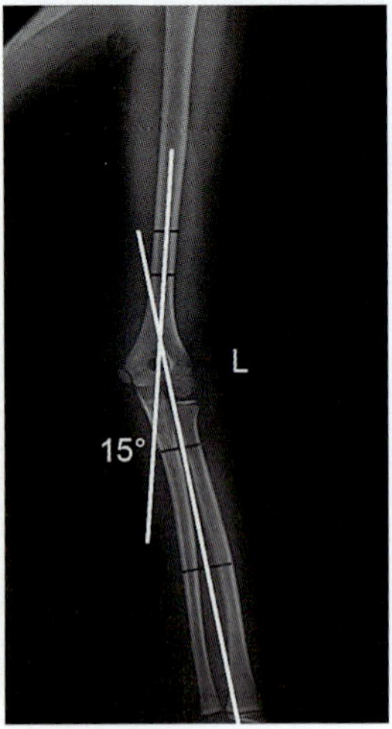

Fig. 2.13: Humerus–elbow–wrist angle.

- *Baumann angle*: It is measured in pediatric age group on a frontal radiograph with elbow in extension. The angle is formed between longitudinal axis of humerus and a straight line passing through the epiphyseal plate of capitulum. The normal value for Baumann angle ranges between 64° and 81°. However, it is better evaluated by comparing its value on contralateral side which should not differ by >5° **(Figs. 2.14A and B)**.

Fat Pads (Fig. 2.15)

There are three extra synovial fat pads around elbow and are grouped as anterior and posterior.

- *Anterior*: Coronoid fossa fat pad and radial fossa fat pad
- *Posterior*: Olecranon fossa fat pad

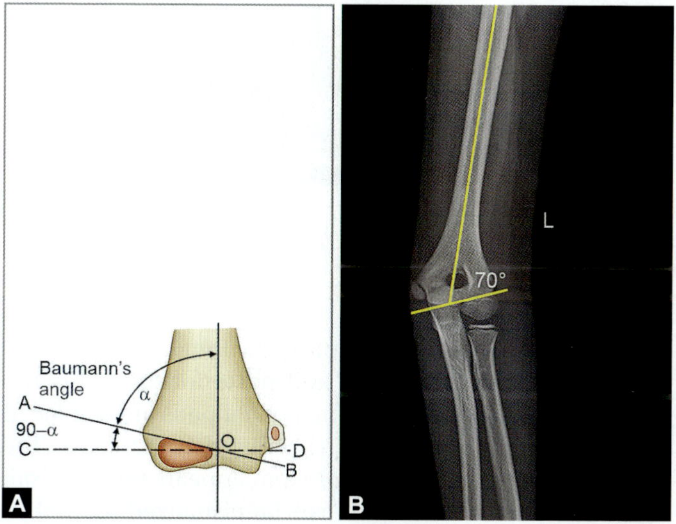

Figs. 2.14A and B: Baumann's angle.

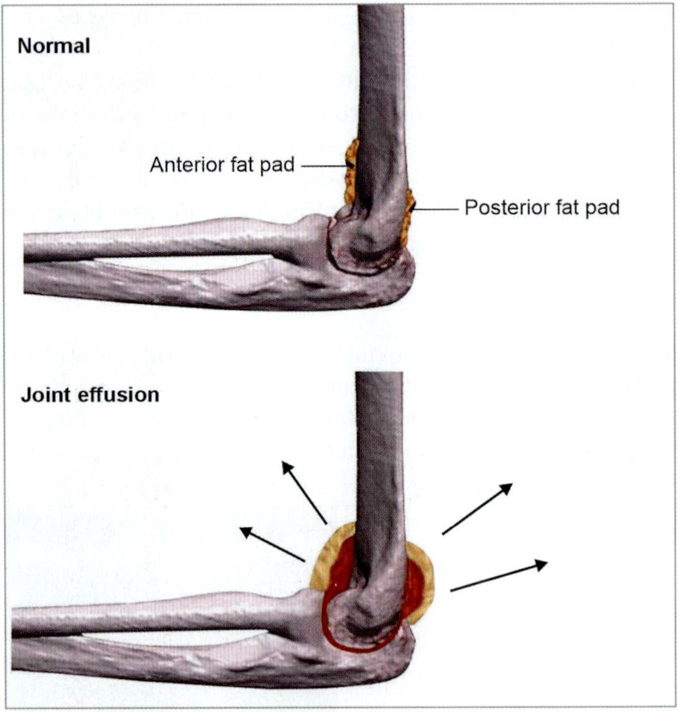

Fig. 2.15: Fat pads.

In a normal lateral view of elbow, only a small stripe of anterior fat pad is visible and posterior fat pad is not seen. In a situation of joint effusion, fat pads are displaced and become more apparent (positive fat pad sign). The anterior fat pad protrudes more and appears pointed (sail sign). The posterior fat pad can be visualized as well in the presence of effusion, and if seen is always abnormal **(Figs. 2.16A and B)**.

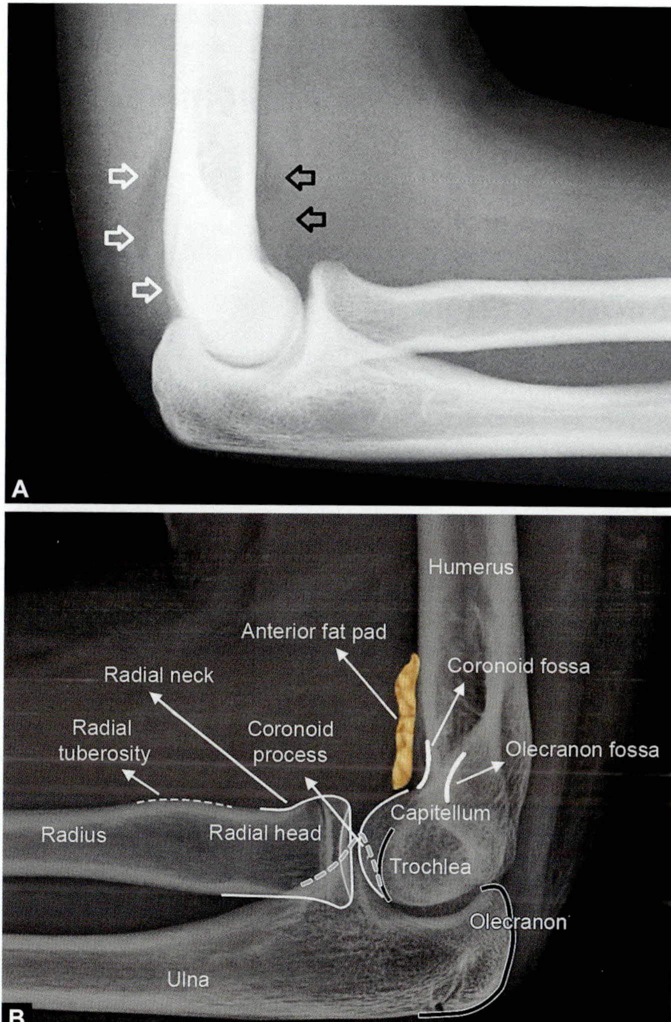

Figs. 2.16A and B: Normal fat pad around elbow and positive fat pad sign on a radiograph.

CHAPTER

3 Biomechanics

INTRODUCTION

Biomechanics is the science between biology and mechanics. The knowledge about biomechanics of elbow is of utmost importance for management of cubitus varus. Still, most of the orthopedic surgeons are not familiar with it.

The elbow joint complex is composed of three bones and three joints enclosed within a fibrous joint capsule. The joints of the elbow complex include the humeroulnar, humeroradial, and the proximal radioulnar joints.

The humeroulnar joint is formed by the articulation between the pulley-like trochlea of the distal humerus and the trochlear notch of the proximal ulna.

The humeroradial articulation is composed of the hemisphere-shaped capitulum on the anterolateral aspect of the distal humerus and the superior aspect, or fovea, of the disk-shaped head of the radius. Because the capitulum lies on the anterior aspect of the distal humerus, the radius articulates with only a portion of the capitulum during elbow extension. Contact between the radius and humerus increases in flexion.

The primary movements that occur at the humeroulnar and humeroradial joints are flexion and extension, which occur about an axis that passes through the center of the trochlea and capitulum and can be approximated by a line through the humeral medial and lateral epicondyles. However, there is also slight medial and lateral mobility (abduction and adduction in the frontal plane) and medial and lateral rotation (about the ulna in the transverse plane).

The proximal radioulnar joint, described as a pivot joint, is formed by the articulation between the rim of the radial head and radial notch or facet on the proximal ulna. The movements that occur in the proximal radioulnar joint, in conjunction with the distal radioulnar joint, are pronation and supination. These motions occur around an axis formed by a line from the center of the fovea of the radial head to the head of the ulna (distal end of the ulna).

This would make it appear that supination and pronation are simple movements that occur when the head of the radius pivots on the ulna and the distal end of the radius glides around a fixed ulna. However, if you observe your own hand pronating around a fixed ulna, you will see your hand moves medially in space.

Pronation, however, can occur without displacement of the hand and without compensation at the shoulder or wrist, as when using a screwdriver. This ability suggests, and several studies demonstrate, that the distal ulna moves radially as the radius rotates around it to keep the hand in a fixed position. This complex movement of both the radius and ulna during pronation and supination provides more evidence that movement in the elbow joint complex is more elaborate than it appears when observing elbow motion grossly.

FUNCTION OF THE ELBOW JOINT COMPLEX (FIG. 3.1)

The joints of the elbow complex participate in a variety of functional activities and conditions. The elbow joint complex enables individuals to place the hand in a variety of positions around the body.

Elbow flexion coupled with supination is used to bring the hand to the body and face to eat, dress, and perform personal care and hygiene, as well as to pull or carry objects. Elbow extension coupled with pronation is used to reach, throw, and push.

Normal or full elbow range of motion (ROM) is reported in the literature by many authors. There is considerable variation in the ROM values reported in different studies; however, in clinical practice, full elbow ROM is typically reported as full extension at 0–5° of hyperextension and full flexion at 135–145°.

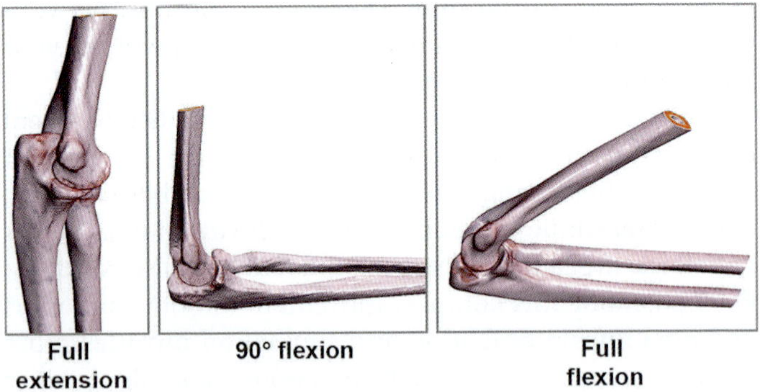

Fig. 3.1: Normal elbow range of motion.

ARTICULATIONS AND ARTHROKINEMATICS

All moving joints must have structure that provides for both mobility and stability. Movement without stability is usually painful, and thus nonfunctional.

Several aspects of the bony structure of the elbow favor stability and control of movement. For example, the distal humerus and proximal radius and ulna fit together in a tongue-and-groove like fashion, making medial and lateral gliding almost impossible. The trochleocapitellar groove between the trochlea and capitulum articulates with the rim of the radial head thus contributing to this stability.

The ridge or crest in the trochlear notch of the proximal ulna tracks in a corresponding groove in the humeral trochlea to limit medial/lateral shifting of the ulna during elbow flexion and extension.

According to Wolff's law, this suggests that the distal humerus sustains its largest loads distally and anteriorly and the trochlear notch receives its greatest loads superiorly and inferiorly. There is also considerable structural congruency between the concave radial head and the hemispherical capitulum.

However, articular contact at this joint is greatly affected by the position of the elbow and forearm.

For example, in elbow extension, the radial head has no contact with the humeral capitulum. During flexion, the radial head moves proximally and contact with the capitulum increases.

Forearm rotation also affects radiocapitellar contact. Supination decreases the radiocapitellar contact, while pronation increases contact.

DOES CUBITUS VARUS CAUSE MORPHOLOGIC AND ALIGNMENT CHANGES IN THE ELBOW JOINT?

The assessment of morphological and alignment changes in the elbow joint can be determined with the help of three-dimensional computer tomography elbow joint.

Morphological Changes

The posterior trochlea, distal part of the lateral capitellum, diameters of the radial head, and articular surface of the ulna in cubitus varus were larger than those of the contralateral normal elbow. In the ulna, the convex portion of the trochlear notch shifted laterally in cubitus varus. Joint alignment in cubitus varus was affected by a shift of the ulna to a more distal and medial position with external rotation and flexion.

Mechanical Axis Changes

In longstanding cubitus varus, medial shift and external rotation of the ulna relative to the humerus can occur, and these joint misalignments may relate to late complications associated with tardy ulnar nerve palsy and tardy posterolateral rotatory instability.

An orthogonal coordinate system is to be considered in the distal humerus. There are three axes perpendicular to each other such as ML_h-axis (mediolateral axis of distal humerus), AP_h-axis (anteroposterior axis of distal humerus), and PD_h-axis (perpendicular to ML-axis of distal humerus) **(Fig. 3.2)**.

- The origin of orthogonal coordinate system is defined as the midpoint between the center of the lateral verge of

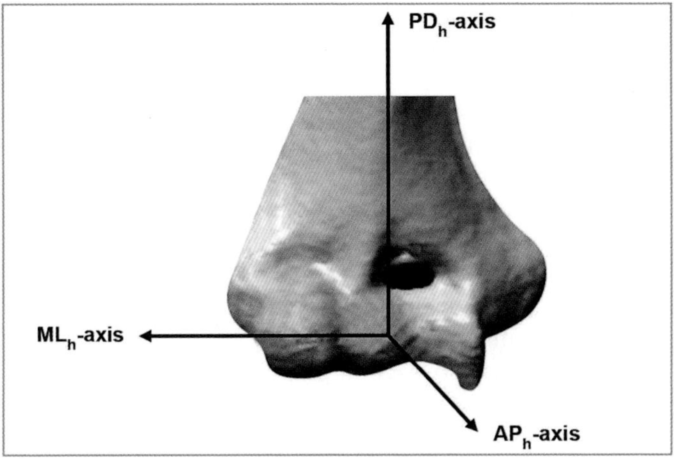

Fig. 3.2: Orthogonal coordinate system of distal humerus.

the capitellum and the center of the medial verge of the trochlea.

- The ML$_h$-axis is defined as the line connecting the center of the lateral verge of the capitellum with the center of the medial verge of the trochlea. The ML$_h$-axis is positive in lateral direction and negative in medial direction.
- The PD$_h$-axis is defined as the line perpendicular to the ML$_h$-axis from the origin in the plane that consisted of the ML$_h$-axis and the midpoint between the bottom of the coronoid fossa and the bottom of the olecranon fossa. The PD$_h$-axis is positive in proximal direction and negative in distal direction.
- The AP$_h$-axis is defined as the line perpendicular to the ML$_h$ and PD$_h$ axes. The AP$_h$-axis is positive in anterior direction and negative in posterior direction.

Similarly, there exists another orthogonal coordinate system in proximal ulna. These are ML$_u$-axis (medial–lateral axis of proximal ulna), AP_u-axis (anteroposterior axis of proximal ulna), and PD_u-axis (perpendicular to ML-axis of proximal ulna).

- The PD_u-axis is defined as the principal axis of inertia of the proximal ulna.
- The AP_u-axis is defined as the line perpendicular to the PD_u-axis and passing the tip of the coronoid.
- The origin of orthogonal coordinate system is defined by intersection of AP_u and PD_u axes.
- The ML_u-axis is defined as the line from the origin perpendicular to the AP_u and PD_u axes.

There are also six sagittal planes, which are parallel to the AP_h–PD_h plane.

The two planes (S1 and S2) divide capitellum in three equal sections, the plane (S3) passing the lateral convexity of the trochlea, the plane (S4) passes the concavity of the trochlea, and the two planes (S5 and S6) divide medial portion of the trochlea in three equal section **(Fig. 3.3)**.

The 3D computed tomography (CT) distal humerus and proximal ulna images of cubitus varus patient:

The posterior part of the trochlea, the distal part of the lateral capitellum, and the diameters of the radial head in cubitus varus were larger than those of the contralateral unaffected elbow **(Figs. 3.4A and B)**. In the ulna, the length of the articular surface in cubitus varus was larger and the convex portion of the trochlear notch shifted laterally on the affected side **(Figs. 3.5A and B)**.

KINEMATICS OF ELBOW JOINT

The movement at the elbow joints is flexion and extension. Movement takes place at three bones—humerus, head

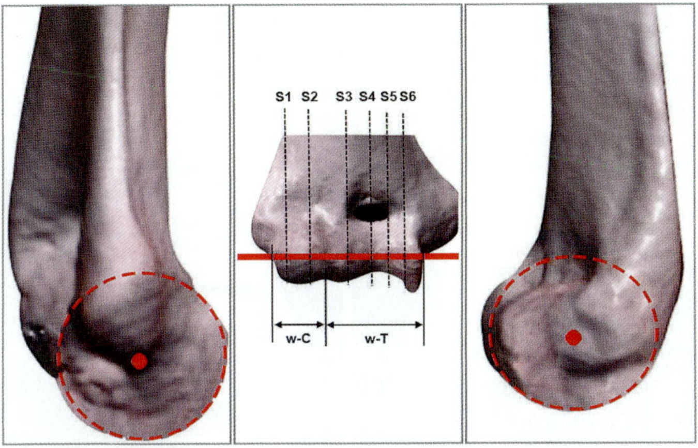

Fig. 3.3: Computed tomography (CT) image.

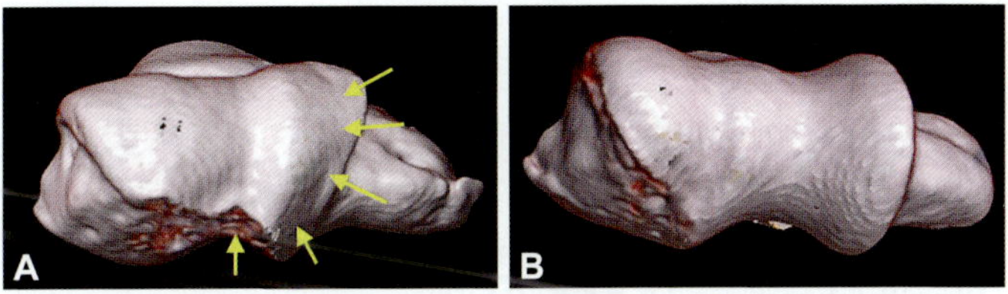

Figs. 3.4A and B: Superimposed 3D surface models show the morphologic changes of the distal humerus in cubitus varus. (A) The posterior trochlea in the affected side was larger (arrowheads). (B) The lateral capitellum in the affected side was larger in the downward direction.

of radius, and olecranon of the ulna. In the humerus, articulation takes place at trochlea and capitellum. Trochlea is tilted 6–8° in the valgus. The movement at the elbow joint is in sagittal plane but since there is 6–8° valgus at the trochlea,

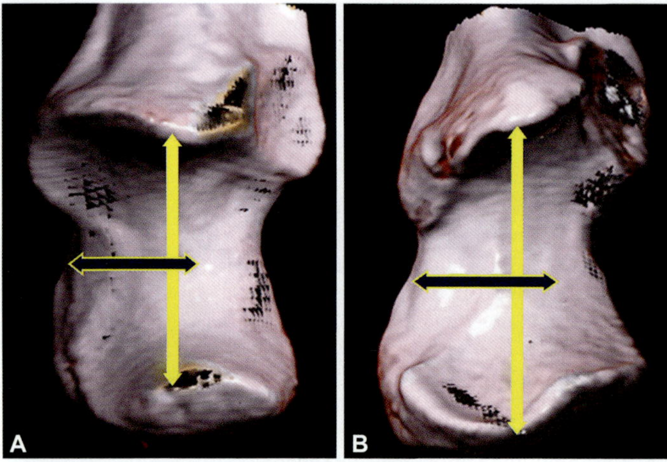

Figs. 3.5A and B: Three-dimensional models show the morphologic changes of the proximal ulna in cubitus varus. (A) The length of the articular surface in cubitus varus is larger. (B) The convex portion of the trochlear notch shifted laterally on the affected side.

the initial movement of the extension is in 6–8° valgus. But gradually extension takes place into the sagittal plane **(Figs. 3.6A to C and 3.7A to C)**.

If you see from the lateral side, radial head moves at the capitellum.

BIOMECHANICS OF THE ELBOW JOINT IN CUBITUS VARUS DEFORMITY

Normally, the elbow joint is in 6–8° valgus and the movement at the elbow joint takes place at the same axis (6–8° valgus). In cubitus varus deformity, instead of 6–8° of valgus, there is a varus deformity at the elbow joint, thus the

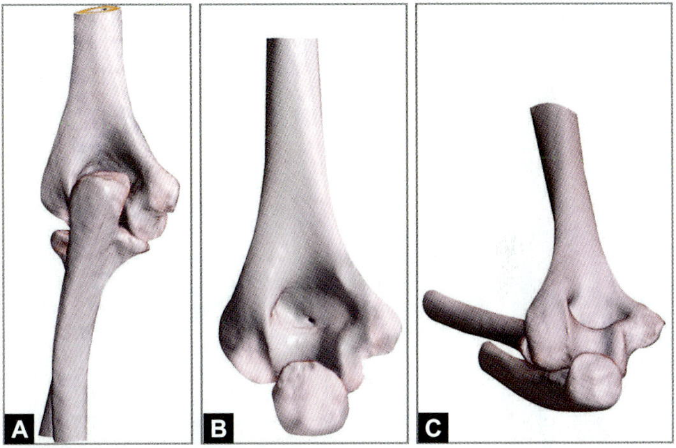

Figs. 3.6A to C: Kinematics of elbow joint. (A) In full extension, olecranon covers the trochlea, making an angle of 6-8°. (B) In 90° elbow flexion, the olecranon will cover half of the trochlea; (C) In full flexion, olecranon covers the anterior portion of the trochlea

lower end of the humerus is tilted into varus. The posterior part of the trochlea, the distal part of the lateral capitellum, and the diameters of the radial head are larger than those of the contralateral unaffected elbow. In the ulna, the length of the articular surface is larger and the convex portion of the trochlear notch shifted laterally on the affected side. This is due to abnormal movement of the elbow joint and leads to damage of the articular surface of the trochlea, capitellum, olecranon, and head of the radius. As the age advances, damage to the articular surface is increased which leads to painful joint. The continuous abnormal movements at the articular surface lead to the damage of the posterior part of trochlea, the distal part of the lateral capitellum, the radial head, and the articular surface of the ulna.

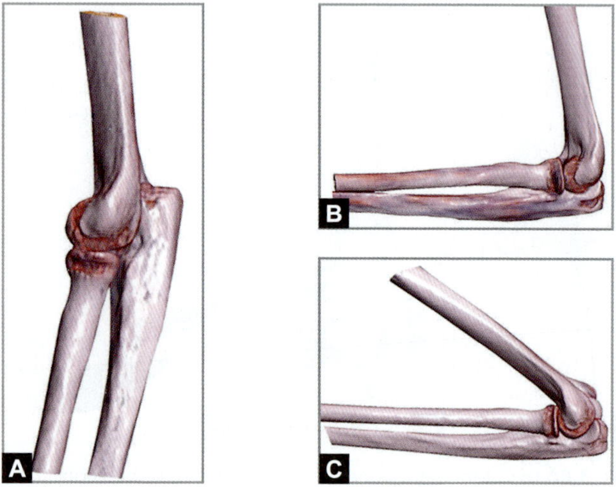

Figs. 3.7A to C: Kinematics of elbow joint. (A) In 90° flexion, head of radius covers the middle portion of the capitellum; (B) In extension, head of the radius cover the lower part of the capitellum; (C) In full flexion, head of the radius covers the anterior part of the capitellum.

KINEMATICS OF JOINT DEFORMITIES

During movement, the point of surface contact between the opposing joint surfaces constantly changes. Even a minor change in alignments of the joints causes great change in joint surface alignments, alteration in motion centers, the ROM, and consequently the stress pattern. Cubitus varus deformity of the elbow is often undervalued as a cosmetic defect only. Careful study will show that acquired cubitus varus deformity, resulting from trauma beyond the age of 7 or 8 years, always causes loss of movement of humeroulnar joint. The author has found that loss of carrying angle up to

0° does not cause any significant loss but for each degree gain in varus angle beyond 0°, there is 2° loss of flexion of the humeroulnar joint. In congenital cubitus varus, the joint surfaces develop adoption to the abnormal longitudinal alignment of the arm and forearm bones and develop its individual motion range and pattern.

CONCLUSION

In elbows with long-standing cubitus varus deformities, the abnormal bone density distribution patterns coincided with most stress distribution patterns, indicating a probable association. We conclude that long-term stress concentration caused by malalignment might lead to altered bone density distribution patterns and that these alterations may develop in the early stages of osteoarthritis (OA) degeneration.

We need to consider correcting malalignment before OA develops and remember that corrective osteotomy in the early stages of degeneration may halt the progression of OA.

CHAPTER

4 Clinical Assessment

INTRODUCTION

Cubitus varus following supracondylar fractures of humerus in children consists of varus, hyperextension, and internal rotation deformities of distal bone fragment of the humerus. Most of the surgeons perform supracondylar osteotomy focused on the correction of varus deformity, not correcting the internal rotation deformity. However, the authors believe that it is also necessary to correct internal rotation and hyperextension deformities of the distal bone fragment in order to obtain clinically and anatomically accurate correction of cubitus varus deformity.

Moreover, preoperative measurement of varus and internal rotation is extremely important. The varus deformity can be measured by carrying angle clinically and radiologically. The internal rotation deformity can be measured clinically and by computer tomography. There are various methods of clinically measuring carrying angle, most common is by goniometer.

MEASUREMENT OF THE CARRYING ANGLE OF THE ELBOW BY GONIOMETER

The bilateral clinical measurement of carrying angle is performed using goniometer. The elbow carrying angle is measured by applying one of the goniometer arm under arm axis and other on the forearm axis with the elbow fully extended and in supine position **(Figs. 4.1A to C)**. The elbows were positioned in extension with forearm supination. All the clinical measurement by the goniometer is examined bilaterally. Certain bony landmarks are marked by making acromion, medial epicondyle, and lateral epicondyle. A line is drawn by connecting acromion

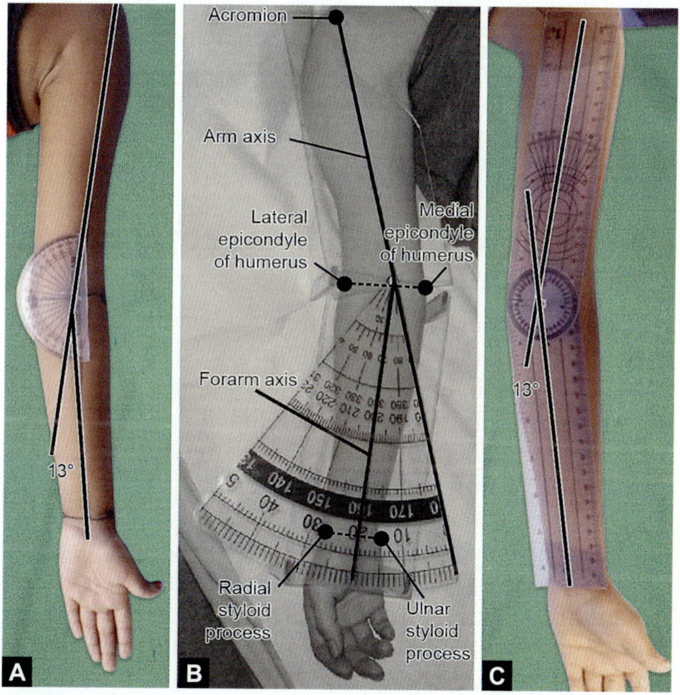

Figs. 4.1A to C: Measurement of the carrying angle of the elbow by goniometer.

and mid of the medial epicondyle and lateral epicondyle. This arm axis was extended downwards. The forearm axis line is drawn from the midpoint of the line joining lateral epicondyle of humerus and medial epicondyle of humerus. This line was connected from the midpoint of the line joining the radial styloid process and ulnar styloid process. The angle between the humeral line and forearm line is measured, this is the varus angle of the affected elbow.

The amount of correction required was calculated by the sum of the varus deformity present and the HEW (humerus-elbow-wrist) angle (carrying angle) of the normal side. The highest value of carrying angle in female gender would be justified by the presence of ligamentous laxity. We believe that the maximum extension of the elbow should contribute to the increase of the elbow carrying angle.

MEASUREMENT OF INTERNAL ROTATION DEFORMITY BY YAMAMOTO

Preoperative measurement of internal rotation deformity is extremely complicated and still there is no simple and reliable clinical method for its measurement. To remedy this situation, Isao Yamamoto developed a useful method of internal rotation that may be applied clinically to correct rotational deformity.

The newly devised method of measuring internal rotation is first made with the subject in an upright position. With the subject bending slightly forward, the upper limb is held at the side and then positioned behind the back with the elbow at 90° flexion and the shoulder held at the maximum extension position. In this position, the midline of the forearm is exposed for inspection by the examiner, who stands behind the subject, applying maximal internal rotation to the subject's upper limb around the long axis

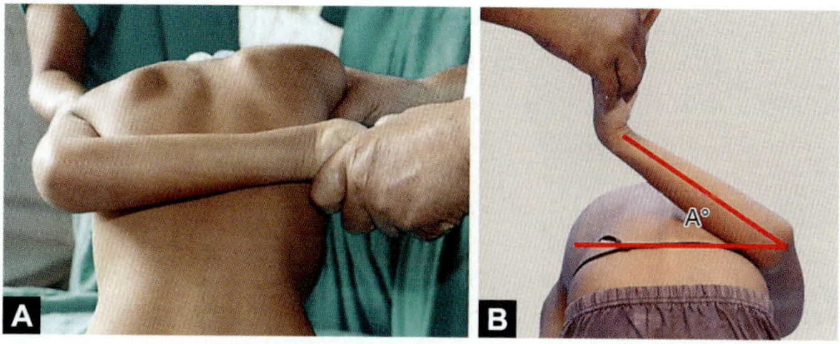

Fig. 4.2A and B: (A) Normal. (B) Cubitus varus.

of the humerus. When no internal rotation deformity of the humerus is present, there is no change in the forearm position. The horizontal plane of the back is parallel with the midline of the forearm **(Fig. 4.2A)**. Conversely, in children with the internal rotation of cubitus varus deformity, a certain abnormal angle is formed between the horizontal plane of the back and the midline of the forearm. This angle is designated as the internal rotation angle **(Fig. 4.2B)**.

Hold patient's elbow as a fulcrum and put the humerus at maximal internal rotation by lifting his hand from the back. In the normal child, the hand cannot be brought up from the back. (B) In case of cubitus varus deformity, the hand is lifted forming an angle (indicated as "A") between the horizontal plane of the midline of the forearm. "A" is assumed as the angle of internal rotation deformity of the humerus, and designated the internal rotation angle **(Figs. 4.3A and B)**.

CARRYING ANGLE

In physiological conditions, carrying angle varies according to age, gender, hyperextension of the elbow, dominant

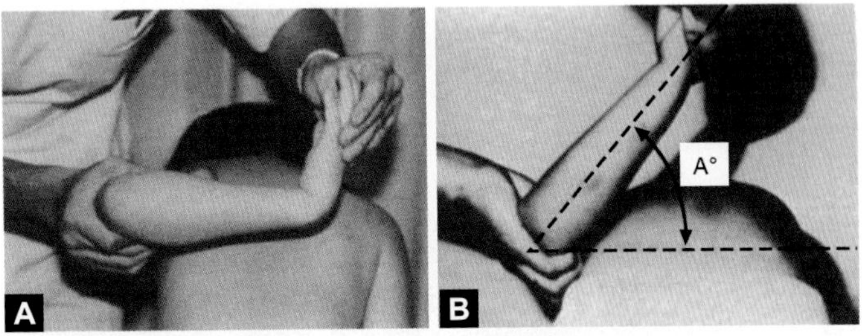

Figs. 4.3A and B: Measurement method of internal rotation angle by authors' method. (A) Have the patient bend forward slightly, setting the forearm behind his back with the elbow flexed 90° and his shoulder hyperextended maximally. (B) In case of cubitus varus deformity, the hand is lifted forming an angle A°.

upper limb, anthropometric characteristics such as height and intertrochanteric distance, and can be measured by simple clinical and radiographic techniques.

The mean value of carrying angle was 12.78° ± 5.35° for the females and 11.20° ± 4.45° for the males **(Fig. 4.4)**.

According to Mall, the axis of the elbow joint is set obliquely at nearly 84° of both the humerus and ulna which is also agreed upon by Jones. Langer was of the opinion that the obliquity of trochlea to the shaft of the humerus is the cause. Kapandji explained that the angle is formed as a result of trochlear groove being vertical anteriorly but on the posterior aspect, it runs obliquely distally and laterally. This results in formation of carrying angle in extension when posterior aspect of the oblique groove makes contact with the trochlear notch of ulna and the angle is marked during flexion when trochlear notch lies on the vertical groove in the anterior aspect. Last suggested that in the ulna a curved ridge joins the prominence of the coronoid and olecranon process which fits the groove in the trochlea of the humerus.

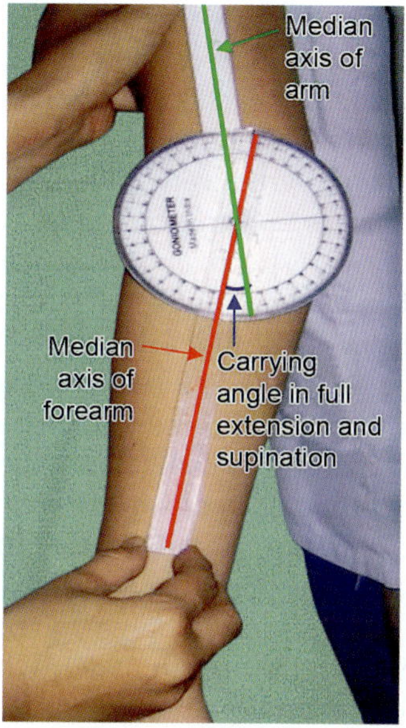

Fig. 4.4: Measurement of carrying angle.

The obliquity of the shaft of ulna to this ridge accounts for most of the carrying angle at elbow. Decker gave the same reason pointing out that the inner lip of trochlea of humerus is a ridge (groove) which is much deeper distally anteriorly so that ulna (with the forearm) is deflected in full extension by this ridge. William et al. considered the medial edge of trochlea of humerus is responsible as it projects nearly 6 mm below the lateral edge and the obliquity of the superior articular surface of the coronoid process which is not set at right angle to the shaft of ulna.

An improvised instrument goniometer is used for measurement of carrying angle. The fixed arm of which could be placed on the median axis of the upper arm, the movable arm adjusted as to lie on the median axis of forearm and the angle read on the goniometer. Bicipital groove, biceps brachii tendon at its insertion, and palmaris longus tendon at the wrist were palpated and marked as anatomical landmarks to demarcate the median axes of the arm and the forearm, respectively. Measurement of carrying angle was taken on the left side as well as on the right side to find out difference on both sides if any.

Difference of the length of forearm of right and left side is statistically insignificant, whereas difference in the length of forearm in the male and female is statistically significant. From the recent study, it is observed that the height and forearm length both are more in males than females. In contrast to this, average carrying angle is more in females than males. We have proposed a new explanation for greater carrying angle in females than in males. When the forearm is pronated, the proximal part angulates. The medial part of the trochlear notch moves more away from the humeral articular surface than the lateral part. Therefore, the medial flange of trochlea is not compressed and grows more than lateral flange. If the height of a person and, therefore, length of ulna is lesser, then because of shorter lever arm, the proximal end has to angulate more in order to bring the hand in pronated position for routine work. Therefore, in a shorter person, the medial part of trochlear notch of ulna goes more away from the medial flange of trochlea which can now grow more than in a person with longer forearm, leading to greater carrying angle. The carrying angle develops in response to the pronation and is dependent on the length of the forearm bones, greater the length of the forearm bone lesser is the angulation of proximal articulation of proximal articular surface, therefore lesser is the carrying angle. From the present study, it is clear that the height and length of the forearm are directly related to each other. Distal part of the humerus particularly trochlea and proximal part of the ulna play major role in the causation of carrying angle. Carrying angle helps in keeping the forearm away from the side of the pelvis when the upper limb swing during walking is also wrong. The carrying angle is only formed when the forearm is fully supinated and extended at elbow. It disappears in pronation or flexion at elbow. Therefore, if the carrying angle is not present and does not help in any way in keeping the forearm away from the side of the pelvis during walking.

THREE-POINT RELATIONSHIP OF ELBOW

The olecranon, lateral, and medial epicondyle form a near equilateral triangle in 90° flexion at elbow. In disruption of elbow joint, the measurements are altered and can be interpreted as below **(Fig. 4.5)**:

- *Decreased length of medial limb of triangle*: Posteromedial dislocation, medial rotation of fractured fragment
- *Decreased length of lateral limb of triangle*: Posterolateral dislocation, lateral rotation of fractured fragment
- *Increased length of medial limb of triangle*: Fractured medial epicondyle/condyle
- *Increased length of lateral limb of triangle*: Fractured lateral epicondyle/condyle
- *Increased base (interepicondylar distance)*: Malunited fracture intercondylar humerus

In cubitus varus, the three-point relationship is maintained.

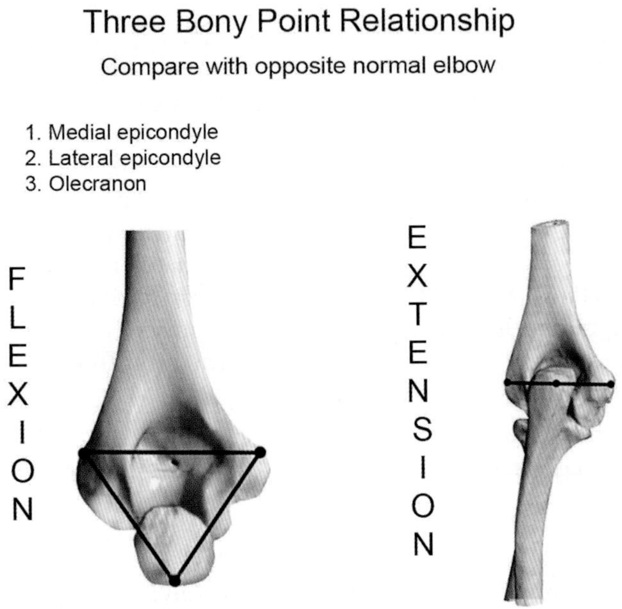

Fig. 4.5: Three-point bony relation of elbow.

CHAPTER

5 Measurement of Radiographic Parameters

HUMERUS–ELBOW–WRIST ANGLE (FIG. 5.1)

The humerus-elbow-wrist (HEW) angle is the angle between the longitudinal axis of the humeral shaft and a line passing through the midpoints of two transverse lines across the forearm. The proximal line is drawn at the level of the radial tuberosity, and the distal line is made at the level of the top of the radial bowing.

The mean HEW angle is 12° (Range: 1–24°). In 1984, Oppenheim et al. first reported on the measurement of the HEW angle with use of full-view radiographs of the humerus and forearm. In that report, the distal transverse line of the forearm is drawn around the distal part of the radius. In 2005, Kim et al. modified the measurement methods by using only radiographs of the elbow. They drew the distal transverse line more proximally, around the top of the radial bowing. Many other studies have evaluated the HEW angle with use of radiographs of the elbow. We believe that it is not practical to routinely make full-view radiographs of the humerus and forearm in the course of postoperative evaluation of an elbow injury. Therefore, we evaluated the HEW angle with the modified methods described by Kim et al.

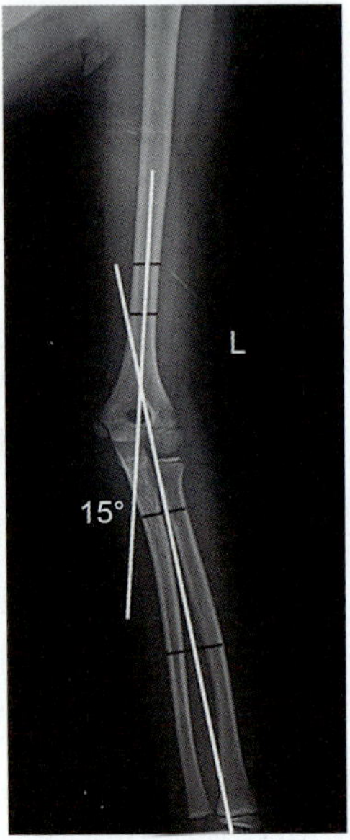

Fig. 5.1: Radiograph illustrating the humerus–elbow–wrist angle.

CARRYING ANGLE

The carrying angle is the angle between the longitudinal axis of the humeral shaft and the longitudinal axis of the shaft of the ulna. The axis of the ulnar shaft is determined by a line passing through the midpoints of two transverse lines (one proximal and one distal). The proximal line is drawn at the level of the olecranon, and the distal line is drawn at the level of the radial tuberosity **(Figs. 5.2A and B)**.

Measurement methods for the carrying angle and the Baumann angle have limitations. Generally, radiographic measurement of the carrying angle is defined by the axes

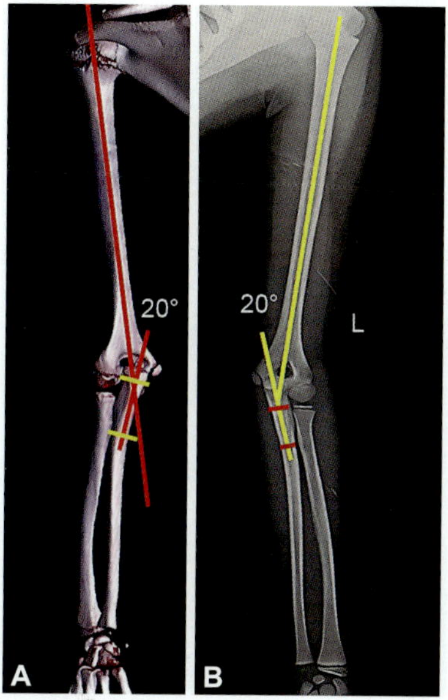

Figs. 5.2A and B: Radiograph illustrating carrying angle between humerus and proximal part of ulna: (A) Computed tomography scan and (B) X-ray.

of the shafts of the humerus and ulna **(Figs. 5.3A and B)**. Because the ulnar shaft is complicated by the S shape of the ulna, definition of the axis of the ulnar shaft is different for each investigator. Different investigators have used the proximal part of the ulna, the diaphysis of the ulna, or the midline between the central points at two locations along the ulna, whereas others have provided no clear definition. Therefore, the reported value of the carrying angle varies according to the definition.

The average of the elbow carrying angle is 12.78° ± 5.35° for females and 11.20° ± 4.45° for males.

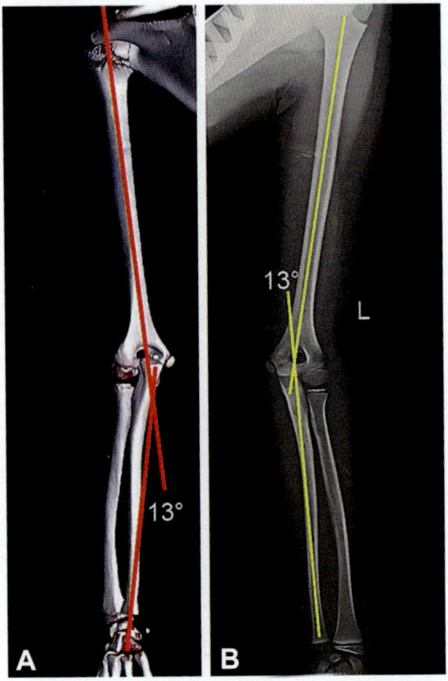

Figs. 5.3A and B: Radiograph illustrating carrying angle between the humeral shaft and diaphysis of ulna shaft: (A) Computed tomography scan and (B) X-ray.

BAUMANN ANGLE

The Baumann angle is the angle between the longitudinal axis of the humeral shaft and a line along the open capitellar physis **(Fig. 5.4)**.

The mean Baumann angle is 71.1° (Range: 56–86°). The Baumann angle is defined by the axis of the humeral shaft and a line along the capitellar physis. Some investigators have doubted the reliability of the Baumann angle because of the difficulty of identifying capitellar growth and distal humeral osseous landmarks. Other authors have indicated that the metaphyseal border is too irregular in

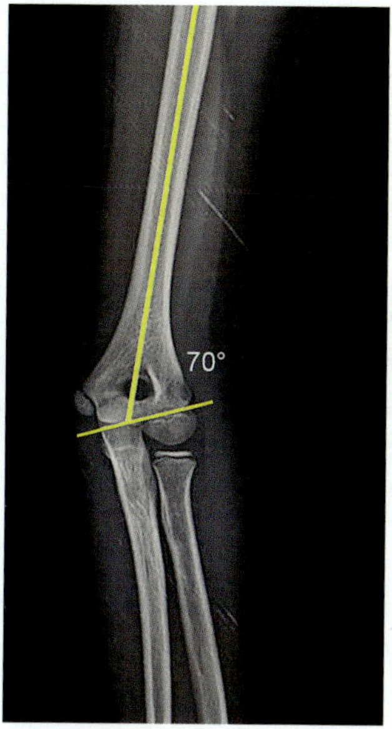

Fig. 5.4: Radiograph illustrating the Baumann angle.

early adolescence, which can alter the measurement of the Baumann angle.

To our knowledge, no previous studies have evaluated the association between the HEW angle and the carrying angle. It is well known that the normal carrying angle ranges from 0° to 25°. An increasing angle represents valgus alignment, and a decreasing angle represents varus alignment. The present study provides evidence that the HEW angle is significantly associated with the carrying angle and is about 3° smaller than the carrying angle. This finding suggests that the HEW angle also can be used to evaluate valgus or varus angulation of the elbow.

PROMINENCE OF LATERAL CONDYLE INDEX

We calculated the lateral condylar prominence index (LCPI) to evaluate objectively preoperative and postoperative amounts of lateral condylar prominence. The LCPI is calculated on the affected side as the difference between the measured medial and lateral widths of the bone from the longitudinal mid humeral axis, and is expressed as a percentage of the total width of the distal humerus to minimize errors from magnification and variation of the size of individual humeri (AB e BC/AC _ 100).

The LCPI is calculated on the affected side as the difference between the measured medial and lateral widths of the bone from the longitudinal mid humeral axis and is expressed as a percentage of the total width of the distal humerus to minimize errors from magnification **(Fig. 5.5)**. The lateral prominence index (LPI) = (AC – BC) × 100/AB.

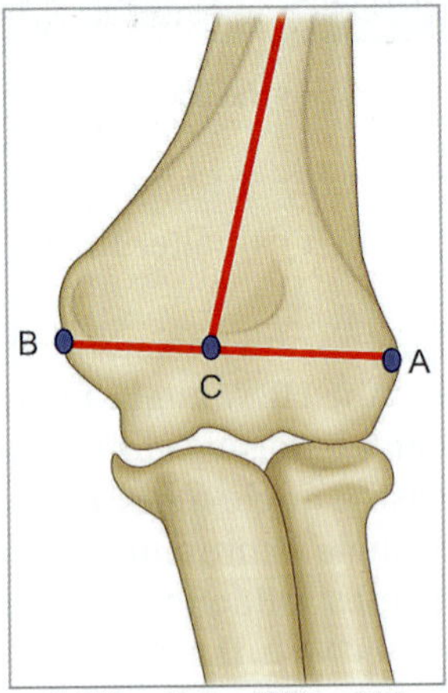

$$(LPI) = \frac{(AC - BC) \times 100}{AB}$$

Fig. 5.5: The lateral prominence index (LPI) = (AC – BC) × 100/AB.

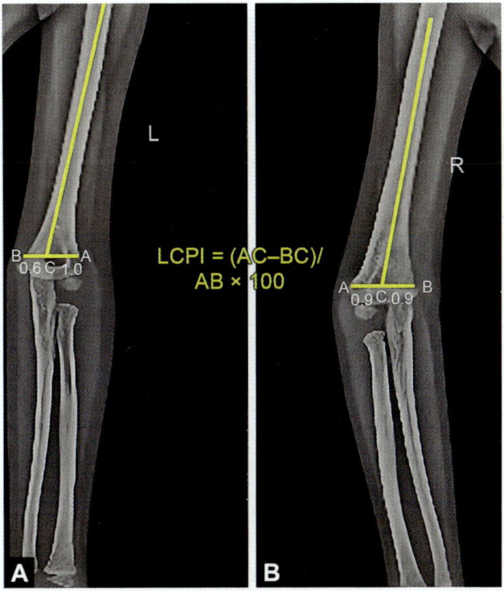

Figs. 5.6A and B: A—lateral prominence; B—medial prominence; C—the cross-link between a line connecting AB, and the longitudinal mid-humeral axis.
Left side: AC = 1.0, BC = 0.6, AB = 1.6 Right side: AC = 0.9, BC = 0.9 AB = 1.8
LCPI = (1.0 – 0.6)/1.6 × 100 = 25% LCPI = (0.9 – 0.9)/1.8 × 100 = 0%

There is usually a slight medial prominence, making the LPI predominantly negative **(Fig. 5.6)**.

TEMPLATING

The purpose of the corrective osteotomy is to produce an elbow joint with a final appearance closely similar to that of the unaffected side. Before planning, radiographs of both upper extremities are taken in the same position with the elbow joints fully extended and the forearms fully supinated. The radiograph of the affected side is then traced **(Fig. 5.6)**. The traced forearm is superimposed on top of the reversed radiograph of the unaffected forearm, and the unaffected humerus is traced. The angle between the central axes of both the affected and the unaffected side is the angle of correction **(Figs. 5.7A to C)**. The angle of correction is copied onto a card in form of a triangle with two equal limbs and with several marks in both limbs at equal distances. The planned triangle is cut out and sterilized **(Figs. 5.7A to C)**.

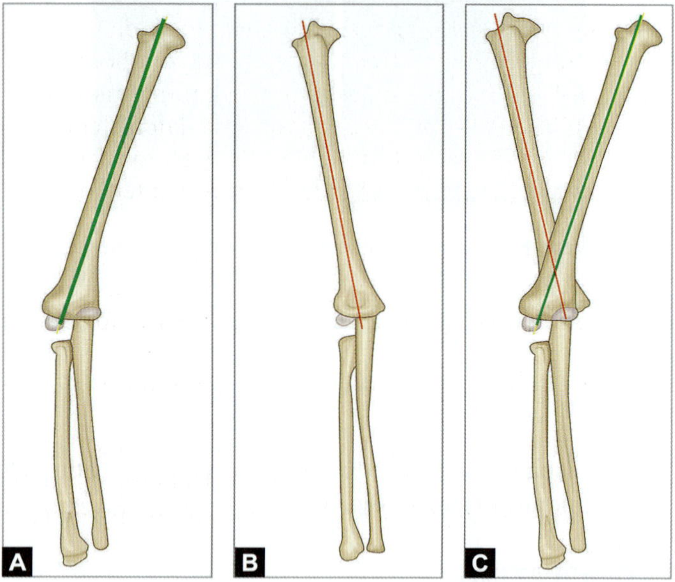

Figs. 5.7A to C: (A) The radiograph of the affected side is first traces (B) The reversed radiograph of the unaffected forearm (C) The affected side is superimposed over the unaffected side, and the angle between the central axes of both the affected and the unaffected side is the angle of correction

CHAPTER

6 Preoperative Planning

INTRODUCTION

Preoperatively, the angle of correction should be calculated clinically by measuring the carrying angle and radiologically, from anteroposterior (AP) and lateral X-rays of both upper limbs. AP radiograph is assessed for humerus–elbow–wrist (HEW) angle of both elbows and lateral condylar prominence. The lateral radiograph is used to record the relationship of the anterior humeral line to capitellum in the sagittal plane (hyperextension).

The amount of correction required is calculated by the sum of the varus deformity present and the HEW angle of the normal side. For example, the varus deformity of the affected elbow is 15° and carrying angle of normal elbow is 11°. The total amount of correction needed is 26° **(Figs. 6.1 to 6.3)**.

Before correction, extension and flexion range of the elbow of both sides is measured. After calculating the angle of correction, preoperative construction of the frame is to be done.

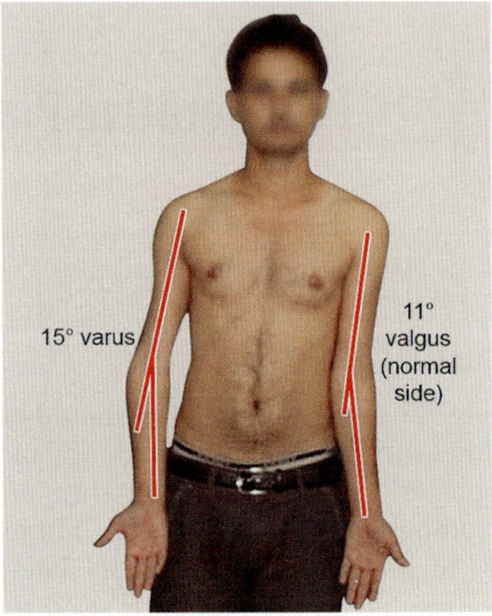

Fig. 6.1: Normal carrying angle 11°, varus deformity 15°.
Note:
Preoperative clinical photos:
The carrying angle of the affected elbow is 15° varus
The carrying angle of normal elbow is 11° valgus
Angle of correction = 15° + 11° = 26°

CONSTRUCTION OF FRAME FOR CUBITUS VARUS CORRECTION

Two-half rings of appropriate size are connected on one side with nut and bolt **(Figs. 6.4 and 6.5)**.

Similarly, the other side is connected to make a full ring. In similar way, same size of the two half-rings is taken to make another full ring. These two full rings are temporarily stabilized by two threaded rods **(Figs. 6.6 and 6.7)**.

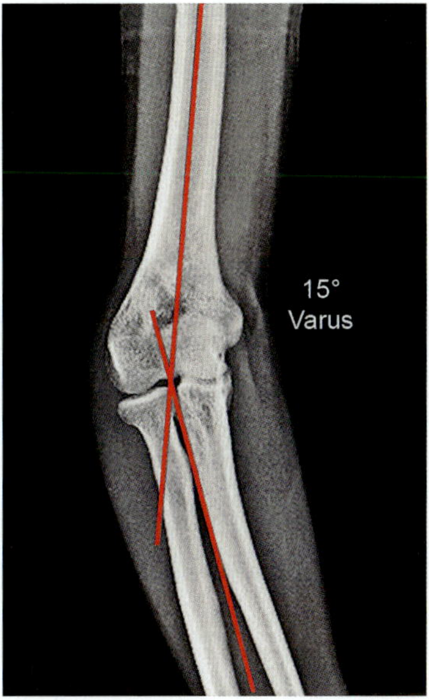

Fig. 6.2: Varus deformity 15° on radiograph.
Note:
Radiographic parameters: The humerus–elbow–wrist (HEW) angle of the affected elbow is 15° varus

Nuts and bolts at the junction of both proximal and distal rings are removed and two male hinges are connected at the junction of distal ring, one on either side **(Figs. 6.8 and 6.9)**.

Similarly, two-hole plates are connected at the junction of proximal half ring. Now, both rings are connected with threaded rods, proximal ring with two-hole plates and distal ring with one-hole male hinges **(Figs. 6.10 and 6.11)**.

A bolt along with a bush is attached to the male hinge **(Fig. 6.12)**.

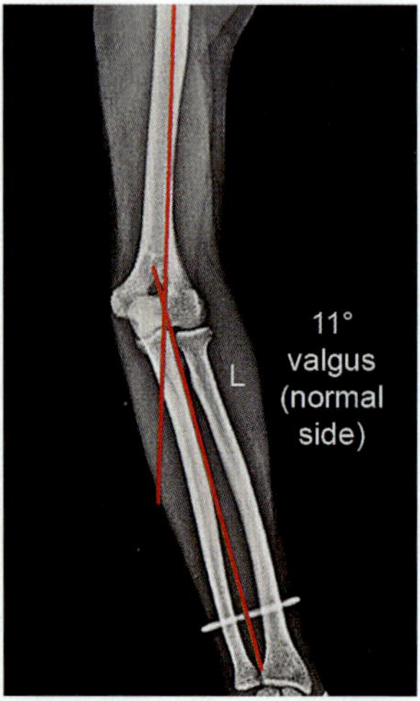

Fig. 6.3: Normal carrying angle 11° on radiograph.
Note:
Radiographic parameters:
The humerus–elbow–wrist (HEW) angle of the normal elbow is 11° valgus
Total angle of correction required will be:
15° + 11° = 26°

Two female hinges are attached to 18-cm threaded rods **(Fig. 6.13)**.

These threaded rods with female hinges are connected to the two-hole plate proximally and one-hole male hinge distally with "30-mm bolt and bush." This hinge is called juxta-articular hinge. The juxta-articular hinges are tightened **(Figs. 6.14 and 6.15)**.

Temporary threaded rods are removed. 90° hinges/twisted plates are placed on medial side of proximal and distal rings for attaching motor distraction rod **(Figs. 6.16 and 6.17)**.

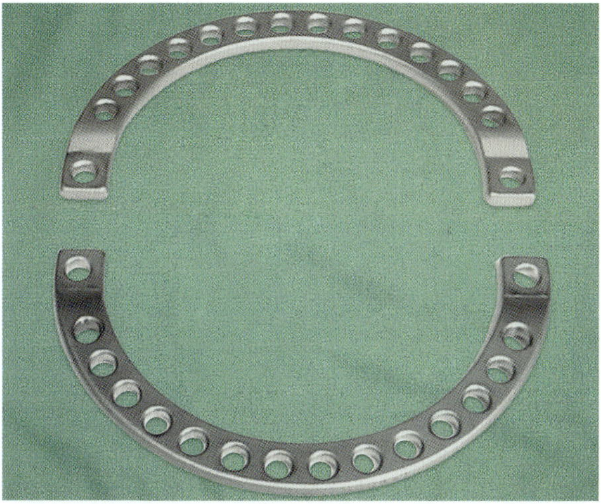

Fig. 6.4: Two half-rings of appropriate size.

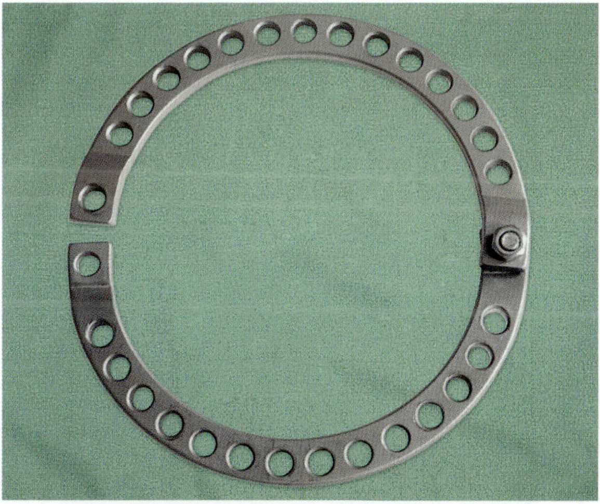

Fig. 6.5: Two half-rings are connected on one side with nut and bolt.

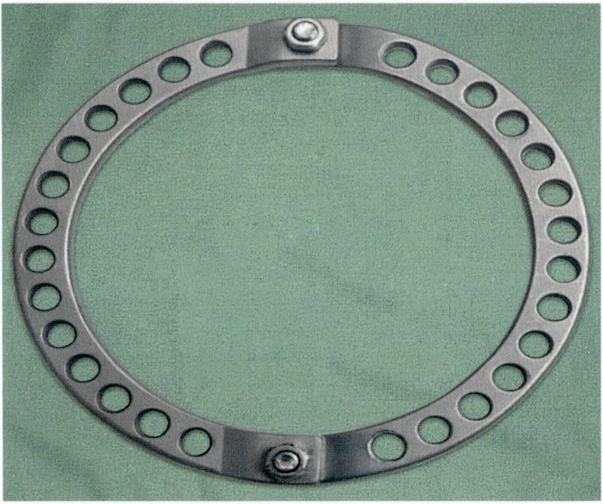

Fig. 6.6: The other sides of the joints of the rings are connected with nut and bolt.

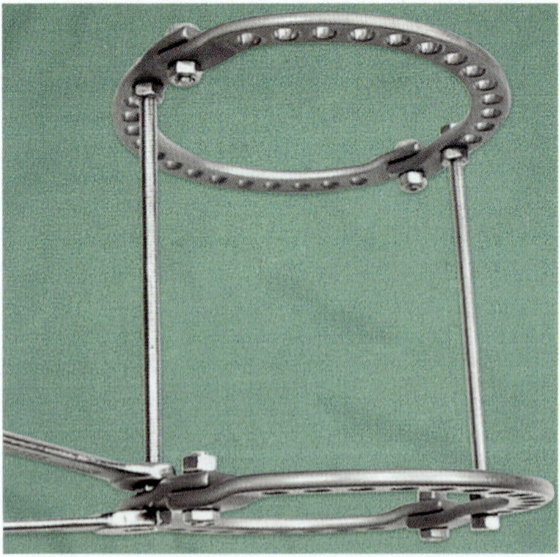

Fig. 6.7: Two full rings are connected by two threaded rods.

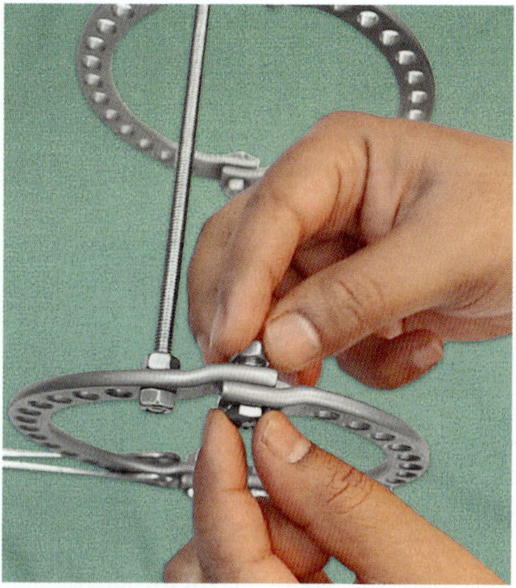

Fig. 6.8: Nuts and bolts are removed at the junction of rings.

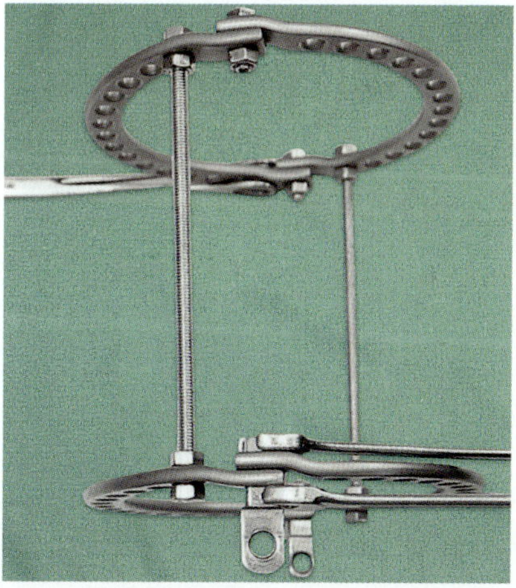

Fig. 6.9: Male hinges are connected at the junction of distal ring.

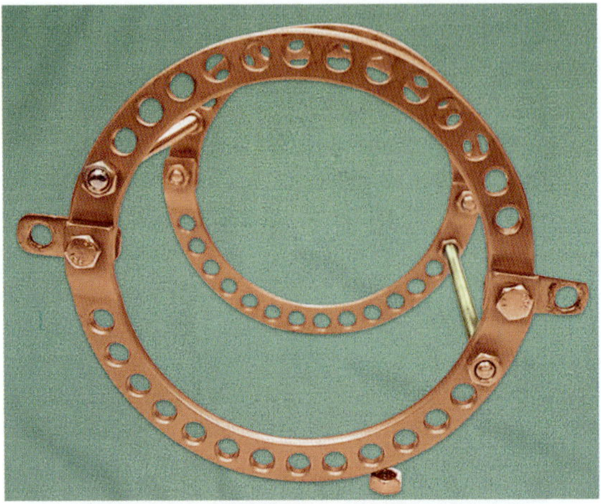

Fig. 6.10: Two-hole plates are connected at the junction of proximal ring.

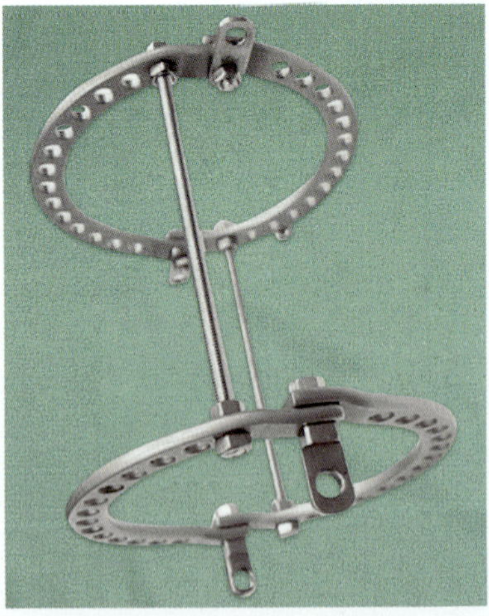

Fig. 6.11: Both rings connected with threaded rods, one-hole male hinge at distal ring and two-hole plates at proximal ring.

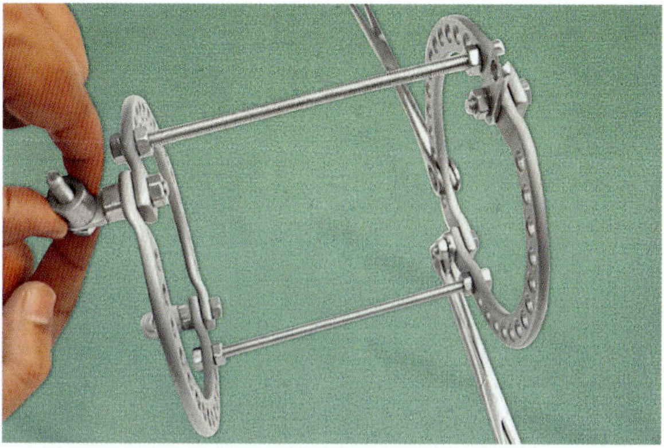

Fig. 6.12: Bolt with bush is attached to the male hinge.

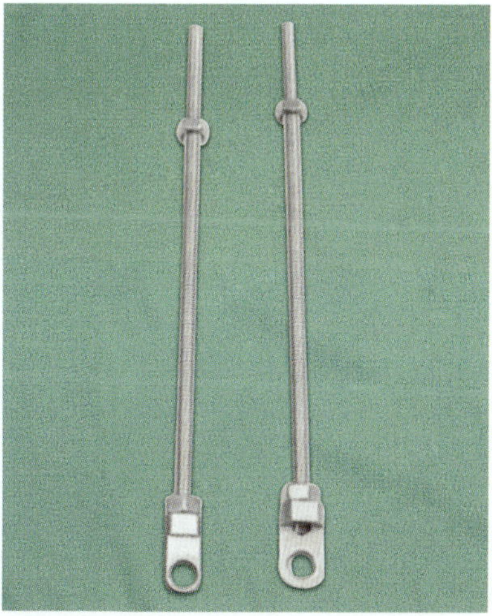

Fig. 6.13: Female hinge is attached to threaded rod.

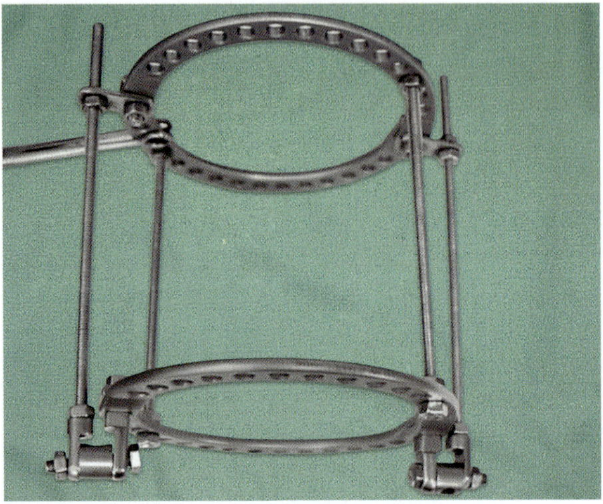

Fig. 6.14: Juxta-articular hinge is made.

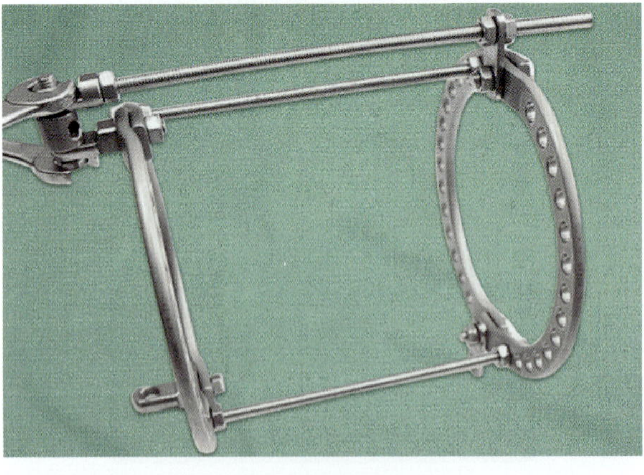

Fig. 6.15: Juxta-articular hinges are tightened.

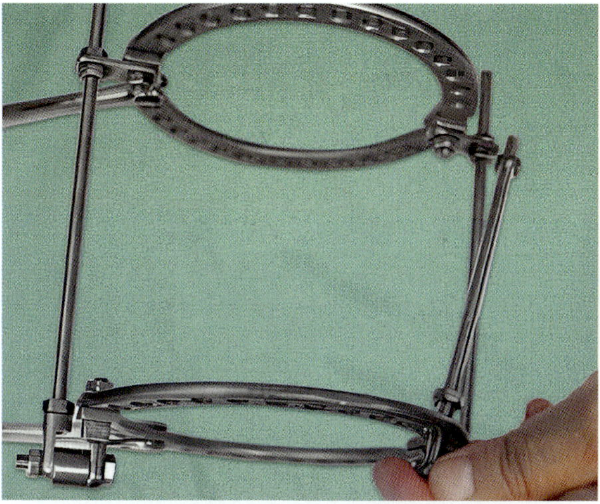

Fig. 6.16: Temporary threaded rods are removed.

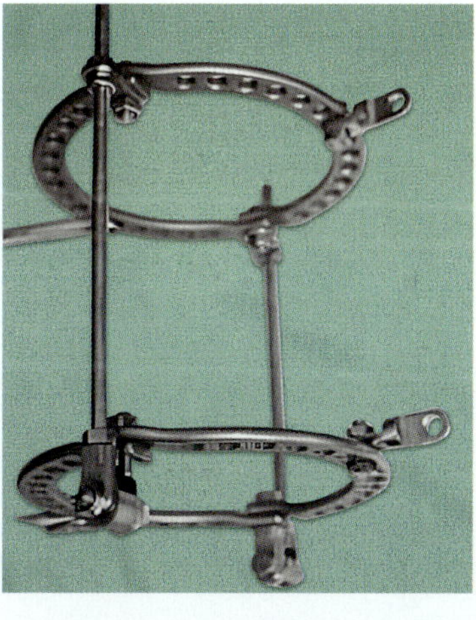

Fig. 6.17: 90° hinges/twisted plates are placed on medial side.

Two male hinges are connected to 90° hinges. Male hinges of proximal and distal rings are connected by threaded rod. This will act as a motor unit **(Figs. 6.18 and 6.19)**.

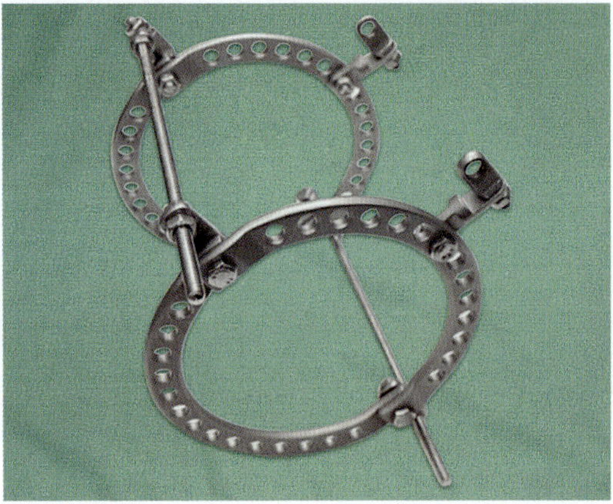

Fig. 6.18: Two male components of hinges are connected to 90° hinges of the twisted plates.

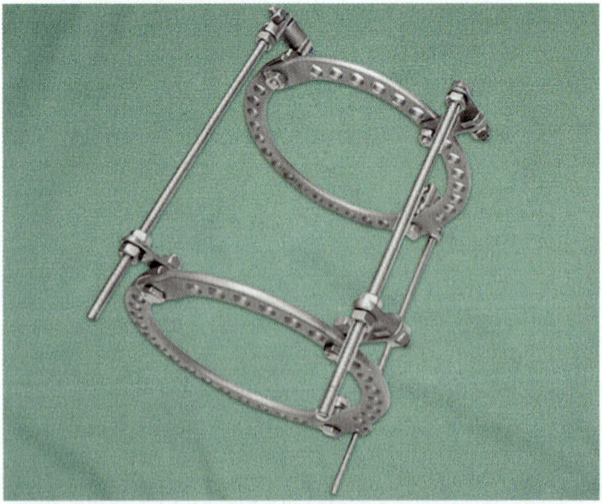

Fig. 6.19: Male hinge of proximal and distal rings are connected by threaded rod.

Nut at male hinge of motor unit of distal ring is loosened. Nut at juxta-articular hinges is loosened. Distal ring is angulated according to the angle of deformity correction and frame is applied over the arm **(Figs. 6.20 and 6.21)**.

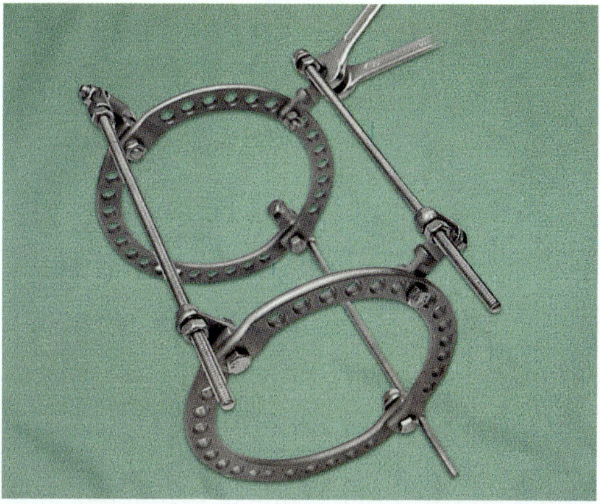

Fig. 6.20: Nut at male hinge of motor unit at distal ring is loosened.

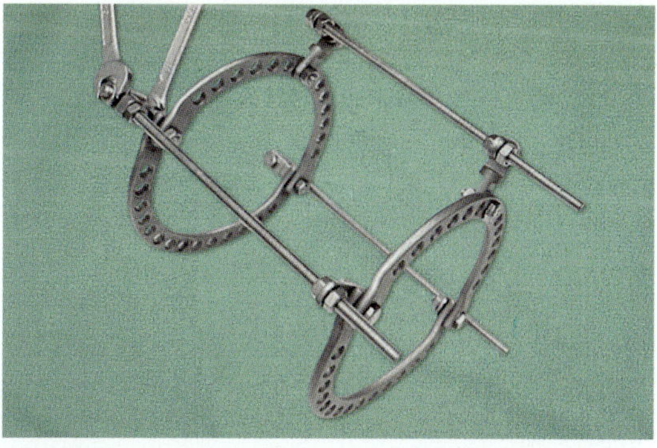

Fig. 6.21: Nut at juxta-articular hinges are loosened.

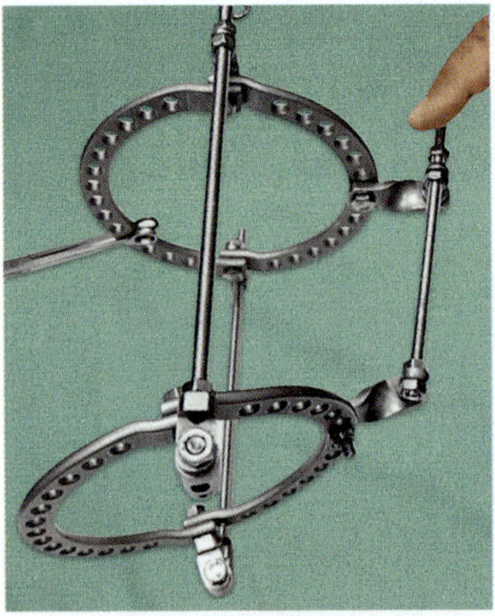

Fig. 6.22: Distal ring is angulated as required on earliar measurement.

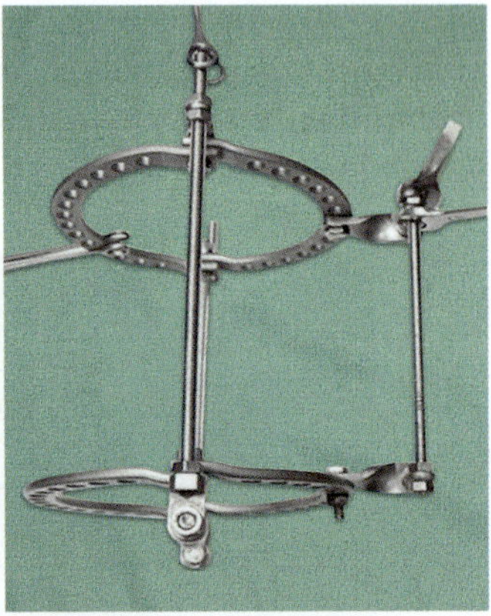

Fig. 6.23: Threaded rod of motor unit is distracted. The deformity is corrected and the rings become parallel.

Threaded rod of motor unit is distracted after doing osteotomy. As the deformity is corrected, both the rings become parallel **(Figs. 6.22 and 6.23)**.

CHAPTER

7 Ilizarov Instrumentation

INTRODUCTION

The Ilizarov apparatus, as an external fixator, distinguishes itself from other monoaxial fixators, because, before it is applied, it must be assembled by the surgeon. In doing so, the surgeon must consider not only the dimensions of the segment being treated, but must also account for numerous other variables.

Many surgeons consider the Ilizarov fixator to be the only elastic and dynamic fixator. But elasticity and dynamics are an intrinsic characteristic of all fixators which reflect the character of the connection between the bone and the fixator. For example, every fixator in which the bone–apparatus connection lies in a straight line, such as monoaxial fixators, allows for dynamic and elastic movement. According to the configuration of the connection, the bone moves in compression but may also move in angulation. This movement, angulation, according to many studies, is defined as "parasitic" and, therefore, can negatively influence the healing of bone.

The real advantage of the Ilizarov apparatus, as an external fixator, is that it uses transosseous wires which minimize this "parasitic" movement (angulation and rotation) without eliminating the elasticity. This, as many biomechanical studies have shown, appears favorable for bone healing.

Elasticity of the fixator does not equate to weakness of the fixator, therefore, it must be constructed "monolith like" as Ilizarov said. And, dynamic does not mean it has to have fewer connection between the bone and frame. Ilizarov, in his work and lectures, always spoke of stability of the apparatus, referring to the bone-fixator connections.

In evaluating Ilizarov apparatus, that is the stability of the fixator, one needs to take into consideration the following variables:

- Rigidity of the assembly
- Connection between the apparatus and the bone
- Intrinsic (or internal) stability of the treated segment

We will now look, step by step, at the various elements that have to be considered when we set out to build our apparatus.

RIGIDITY OF THE ASSEMBLY

The material from which the half rings are made must be extremely solid and allow minimal bending when subjected to the stress of loading and tensioning of the wires.

The steel which is currently used, with a thickness of 6 mm, is considered the best with respect to weight-rigidity-cost. The carbon fiber rings of the same diameter allow for adequate rigidity to loading, but have a tendency to twist if subjected to the stress of wire tensioning; however, with an augmented thickness to 7–8 mm, this problem is resolved.

The diameter of the ring is inversely proportional to the rigidity of the construct. So, the surgeon, who has a choice, should favor the smallest diameter. However, it is recommended that a minimum distance of 2 cm between the soft tissues and the frame be maintained and that this distance be increased to 3 cm where the formation of significant swelling may occur.

The number of rings is directly proportional to the stability of the system. Therefore, when possible, try to construct frames that have two rings per segment. For example, use four rings for a lengthening.

The connection between the half rings is important. With oblique coplanar connections, there is a tendency to twist in the plane of the ring during wire tensioning. Therefore, for a frame in which there is fixation of one segment with only one ring, it is mandatory to use rings with a standard off-set connection. In this configuration, there are fewer number of holes, and therefore much more resistance to stress.

The rings with oblique coplanar connections have to be reserved for that assembly in which one utilizes a block (two rings connected with rods or sockets).

The number of connections between the various rings is directly proportional to the stability of the assembly.

The drawback here is that the more connections that are applied, the fewer the holes that are available for the application of other parts. The correct number of connections for minimal stability is at least four.

Another factor that influences the stability of the assembly depends upon the type of connection between the various rings; for example, a block of two rings connected with a hexagonal socket is much more stable than a block that uses a threaded rod or a threaded rod with conical washers. This allows for "parasitic" angular or rotational motion between the rings.

The stability of the apparatus is inversely proportional to the distance between the rings. So, in a frame constructed for lengthening, where, by necessary, the osteotomy must be performed in the metaphyseal region, it is advantageous to move the intermediate rings closer together.

CONNECTION OF THE APPARATUS TO THE BONE

The diameter of the wire is directly proportional to the stability of the assembly, that is, a larger diameter wire provides more stability.

Normally, in an adult, 1.8-mm diameter wires are used, while in a child or an adult forearm, a 1.5-mm diameter wire is used.

Also, the number of wires used per ring is directly proportional to the stability of the apparatus. The minimum number, in a wire configuration, is two wires per ring. The tension of the wire is also directly proportional to the stability. Normally, a 1.8-mm diameter wire is tensioned to approximately 110 kg, while a 1.5-mm diameter wire is tensioned to about 90 kg. Less tension must be applied to a wire used on a half ring or a five-eight ring (maximum 50 kg) to prevent ring deformation.

Regarding the crossing of the wires, the best configuration is 90° between one wire and other. The larger the angle of intersection, the greater the stability of the basic part (ring and two wires). The stability decreases with a smaller angle, but is relatively sufficient if the final angle is 45°. Below 45°, the stability decreases rapidly in the plane of the obtuse angle of crossing, invariably motion occurs in the other planes.

Twelve years ago, the original Ilizarov apparatus (rings and wires) was modified for the femoral configuration. This was done with the introduction of arches of smaller dimension fixed to the bone with half pins. The half pins were

5-6 mm in diameter. Obviously, this innovation influenced the stability of the whole system (using more rigid materials and greater diameter half pins increased the stability of the system). Pin configuration described by Catagni-Cattaneo (the so called delta pattern) provides better stability with the pins crossing at 60-90°. This configuration is the result of observing other fixator (Hoffman, 1983) along with the clinical experience of the creator of the assembly.

Finally, with regard to the bone fixator connection, one needs to consider the centralization of the bone axis with respect to the central axis of the apparatus. The closer the longitudinal axis of the bone is to the central aspect of the frame, the more stable the apparatus will be. For anatomic reasons (soft tissues), unfortunately, this ideal configuration is difficult to achieve in the tibia while it is more easily obtained in the femur, humerus, and forearm.

INTERNAL STABILITY

Very important, to the stability of the system, is what is more easily defined as internal stability.

In evaluating a fracture or pseudoarthrosis, one needs to first evaluate the surface area of the injury site—the larger the surface area, the better the stability and, therefore, the possibility of allowing weight bearing.

In lengthening a bone, the quality of the regenerate, its diameter, and its maturation determined the intrinsic stability. The better the maturation, the larger the diameter, and the lesser the length of the regenerate, the more stable is the resulting system. One also needs to keep in mind the quality and the quantity of the soft tissues that surround the bone segment in treatment.

And lastly, do not forget the length of the segment treated: in fact, length interferes negatively with the stability of the whole system.

Summary

Variables which are directly proportional to the stability of the system:

- Rigidity of the materials of the rings
- Number of rings
- Rigidity of the connection between the rings
- Number of the connection between the rings
- Diameter of the wires
- Number of wires
- Tension of the wires
- Crossing angle of the wires
- Diameter and angle of crossing of the half pins
- Centralization of the apparatus
- Surface area of the contact between bone ends
- Diameter of the regenerate and its maturation

Variables which are inversely proportional to the stability of the system:

- Length of the connection between the rings
- Length of the regenerate
- Length of treated segment

Now we can look at what variables are controlled by the surgeon:

- Construction of a stable apparatus with enough rings (at least two levels of fixation per each bone segment)
- Enough wires and half pins per each basic part (ring or arch) (two wires per ring or one half pin or one wire and two half pins)

- In regards to the internal stability, it is necessary to have a good reduction of the fracture and adequate surface contact of a pseudoarthrosis. If necessary, use open reduction to optimize fracture reduction. In the nonunion, bone ends may need to be opened and remodeled to optimize surface contact.
- The diameter of the regenerate depends on the level of the corticotomy. The corticotomy must be performed in the metaphyseal region where the bone has a larger cross-sectional area.
- Obviously, for a good regenerate, the corticotomy needs to be accurate. One must not damage the periosteum nor traumatize the bone. Avoid the use of an oscillating saw or aggressive manipulation.
- The maturation of the regenerate can be guided by careful observation and applying a rhythm of elongation that respects the biology of the patient; if there is slow maturation, the surgeon can intervene with an accord on maneuver or in extreme cases of atrophic regenerate, he may add bone graft.

In conclusion, we again review the basics for stable construction of a circular frame:

- Select an appropriate diameter ring
- At least four connections between the level of the rings and point of bone instability
- Two levels of fixation for each injured bone segment
- Monitor the stability of the parts of the fixator frequently, changing the apparatus during treatment as indicated
- Osteotomy at low energy, subperiosteal, percutaneous in metaphyseal region
- Observe closely the regenerate bone with ultrasound and X-ray

ILIZAROV HARDWARE

The components of Ilizarov apparatus can be divided into two categories—a main and a secondary one.

1. The main parts are standard elements used to correct skeletal deformities—wires (with/without stoppers or olives), half pins, full rings, half rings, arches, wire fixation bolts, (cannulated and slotted), pin clamps, and wire fixation buckles.
2. The secondary parts of the fixator consist of the standard elements necessary for the assembly of apparatus. Namely, threaded rods, telescopic rods, threaded rods with slots, connection plates, curved and twisted plates, supports and posts, hinges, washers, sockets, bushing, bolts, and nuts. To assemble the numerous pieces of equipment, various types of wrenches and wire tensioners are needed.

Half Ring

The ring is made-up of either stainless steel with a mechanical resistance greater than 90 kg/mm^2 or carbon composite ring.

It is available in 12 sizes, viz., 80, 100, 110, 120, 130, 140, 150, 160, 180, 200, 220, and 240 mm inner diameter. Hole diameter of 8 mm with clear spacing between holes of 4 mm. Half rings are ledged at the ends to accommodate the other half ring so that the assembled ring is in one plane **(Figs. 7.1 and 7.2)**.

5/8 Ring

It is available in three sizes of inner diameter 130, 150, and 160 mm. Hole diameter and spacing are same as that of

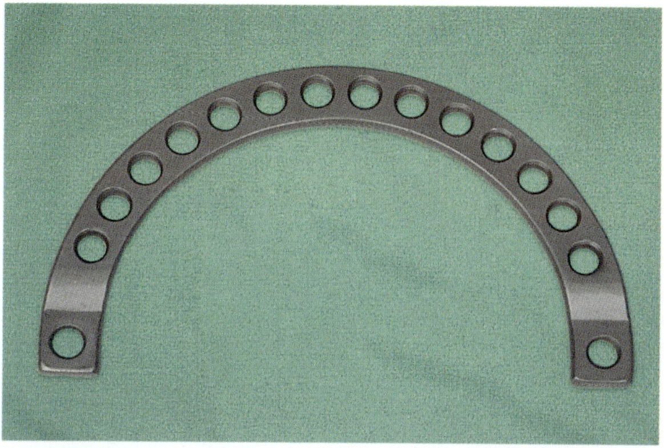

Fig. 7.1: Half ring.

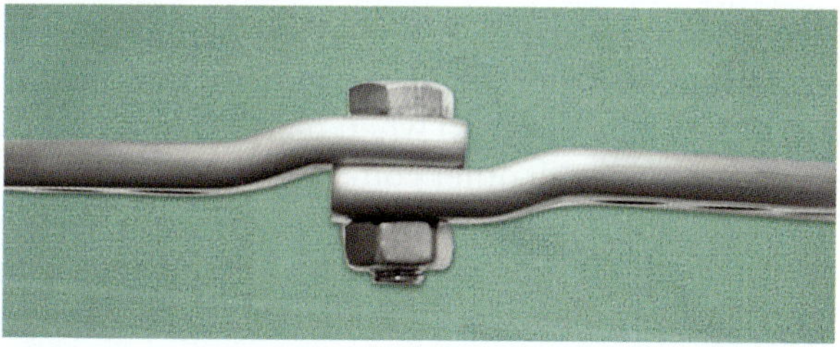

Fig. 7.2: Connected ring.

half rings. It is used near joints to facilitate movement and dressing of open wounds. It is used in combination with another full ring for reinforcement **(Fig. 7.3)**.

Threaded Rod

Threaded rod is of 6 mm diameter with a thread pitch of 1 mm. These are available in lengths of 40, 60, 80, 100, 120, 150, 200,

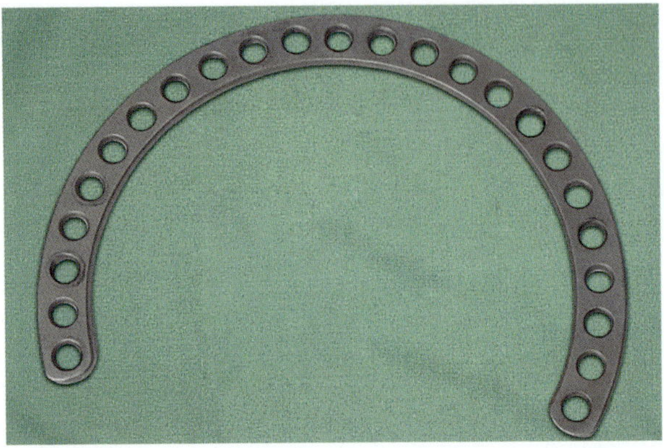

Fig. 7.3: 5/8 ring.

250, 300, 350, and 400 mm, to be used to interconnect rings/arches. Three connecting rods are sufficient to provide the desired mechanical strength when placed 120° apart. Since holes are engaged with other components, it is not possible to maintain 120° spacing and hence four connecting rods are used. Threaded rods can withstand high axial loading but with increased length their stability to resist bending reduces. It is advisable to keep the length of connecting rods not greater than that of the diameter of the rings **(Fig. 7.4)**.

Post

Post is a short plate with 2 to 4 smooth holes of 7 mm diameter and is used as an auxiliary support element for fixing wires/rods/plates at any angle to the main support. They can also be used as locked/mobile joints that can be assembled into multiplanar hinges **(Figs. 7.5A and B)**.

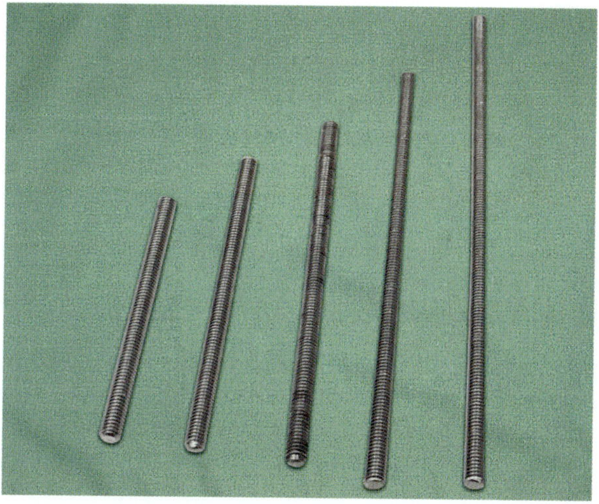

Fig. 7.4: Threaded rods.

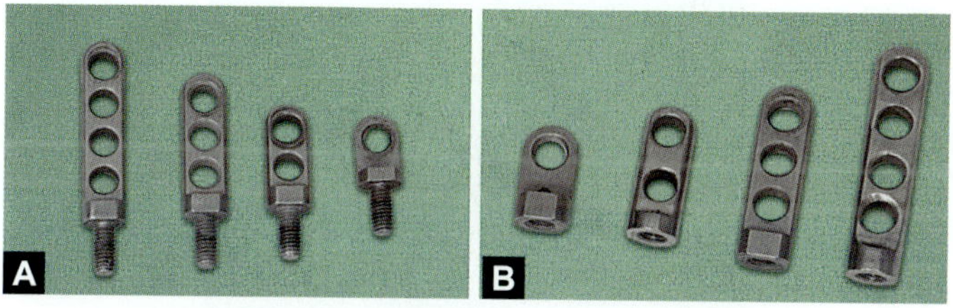

Figs. 7.5A and B: Male and female post.

Posts may be male or female. Male posts are 28, 38, or 48 mm long with 2, 3, and 4 holes respectively. Female posts are 30, 40, or 50 mm long with 2, 3, and 4 holes respectively.

Hinges

Hinge female standard and low profile **(Fig. 7.6)**: These have a supporting base with two flat surfaces for matching standard 10 mm wrench. It has only one hole which is 4 mm thick at base. Low profile half hinges of 30 mm height are also used in multiple planes (hinges have flange on one side).

Construction of hinge **(Fig. 7.7)**
Hinge male standard and low profile **(Figs. 7.8A to C)**

Hinge—90° standard and 90° low profile **(Fig. 7.9)**: In 90° hinges, two flanges are positioned at right angles to the long axis and can be used as a middle component of a two-axis hinge **(Fig. 7.9)**.

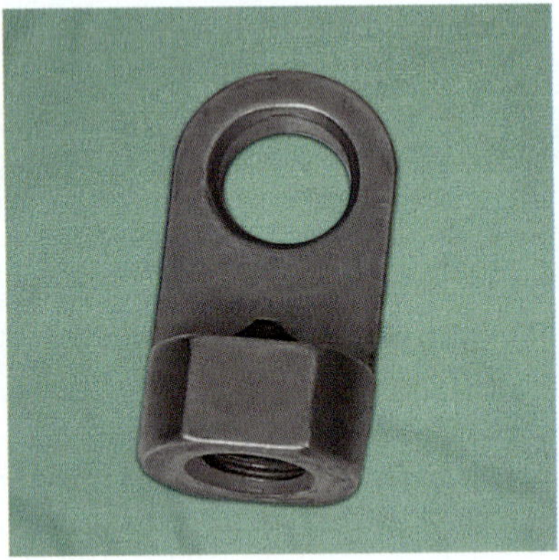

Fig. 7.6: Hinge female.

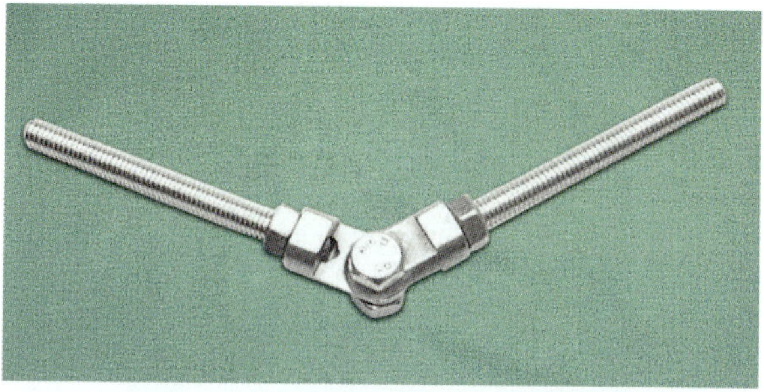

Fig. 7.7: Construction of hinge.

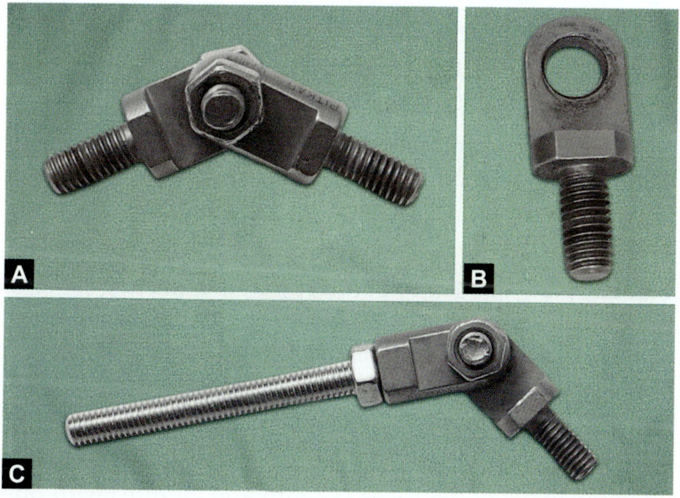

Figs. 7.8A to C: Types of hinge.

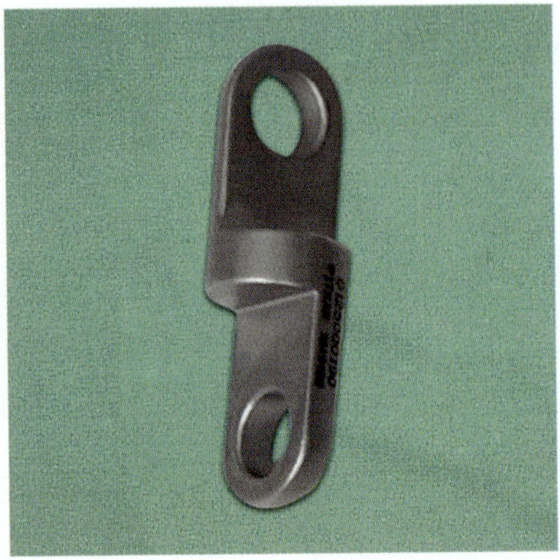

Fig. 7.9: 90° hinge.

Short Connecting Plate

Short connecting plates are available in 9 sizes with 2 to 10 holes. Most commonly used are 2 and 3 hole plates for extension of the main frame **(Fig. 7.10)**.

Twisted Plates

Twisted plate is used to connect long connecting plate to the frame. These plates are used to connect between holes of vertical and horizontal planes. They are of 45, 65, and 85 mm lengths with 2, 3, and 4 holes respectively **(Fig. 7.11)**.

Bushing

The bushing is of two sizes (12 mm and 24 mm) with one and two perpendicular holes. It is short 12 mm cylinder with a smooth unthreaded aperture (7 mm in diameter). It is 1 mm wider than threaded rod. It moves smoothly over the threaded rod. It is also used as spacer **(Fig. 7.12)**.

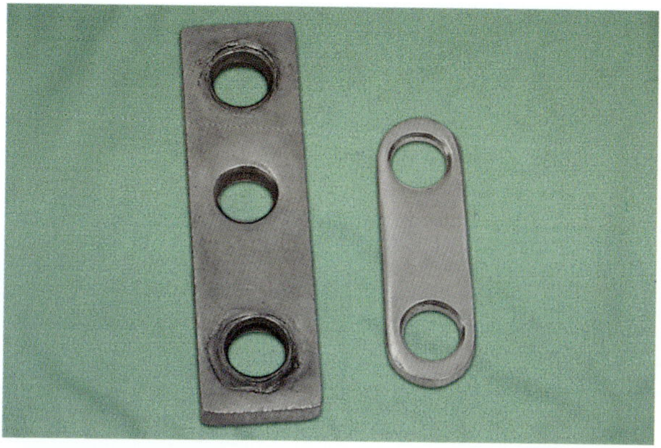

Fig. 7.10: Connecting plates.

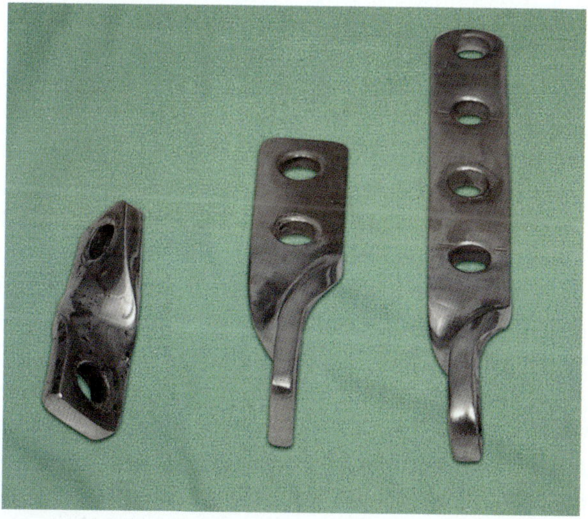

Fig. 7.11: Twisted plates.

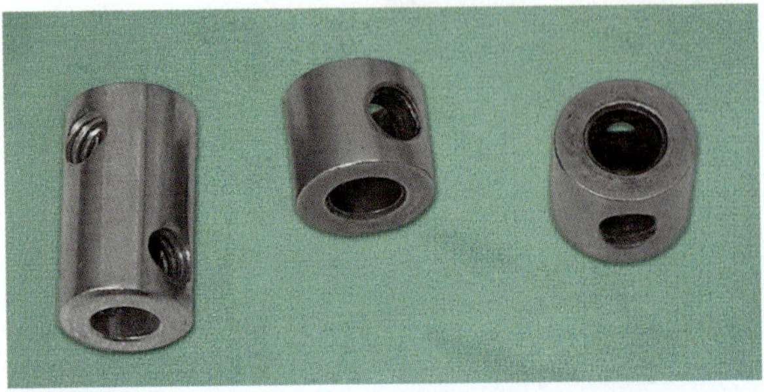

Fig. 7.12: Bush.

Connecting Bolt

It is available in standard sizes of 10, 16, 20, and 30 mm and 4 mm thickness **(Fig. 7.13)**. 10 mm bolts are used only for securing threaded rods and pins through aperture of sockets, bushings, and telescopic rods. It is also used for connecting threaded sockets and bushings to rings/ connecting plates.

- 16 mm bolts are the most commonly used connecting bolts since the thickness of the main components varies between 4 and 5 mm and the thickness of the nuts 5 mm.
- 20 mm bolts are used to connect female hinges.
- 30 mm bolts are used to connect three or more parts.

They can also be used at places to bridge the distance from the rings to pins/wires conveniently.

Nut

Nut is available in thickness of 3, 5, and 6 mm. 3 mm nuts are used only as locking nuts on hinges. 5 mm nuts are used for stabilizing all forms of frame construction. 6 mm nuts are to be used on connecting rods where compression/distraction

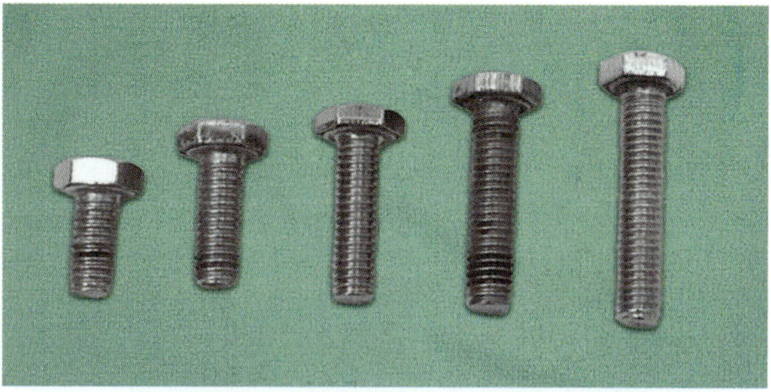

Fig. 7.13: Bolt.

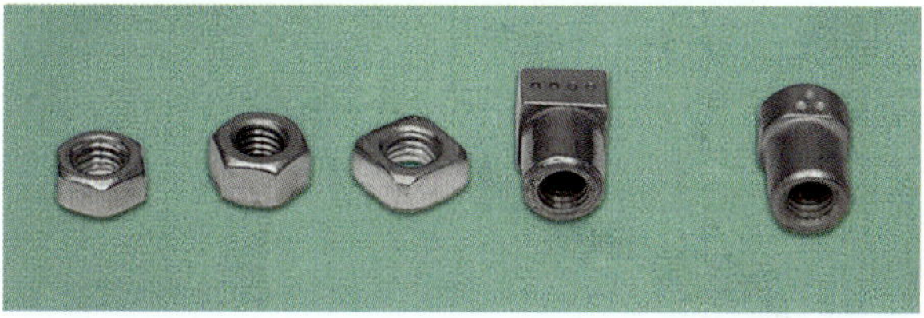

Fig. 7.14: Nut.

is required. These are used at hinges to have controlled motion **(Fig. 7.14)**.

Nylon Insert Nut

Nylon insert nut is used in hinges to perform controlled motion **(Fig. 7.15)**.

Quadrangular Square Head Nut

Quadrangular square head nut is 10 mm long and has a quadrangular head. The head is marked numerically from 1 to 4 or dotted to facilitate rate of lengthening/compression **(Fig. 7.16)**.

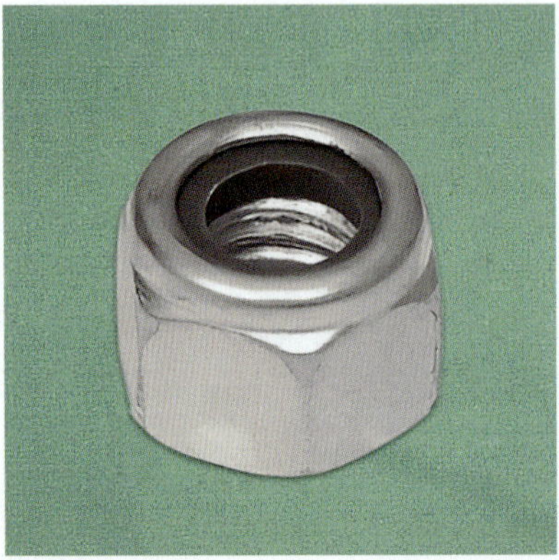

Fig. 7.15: Nylon insert nut.

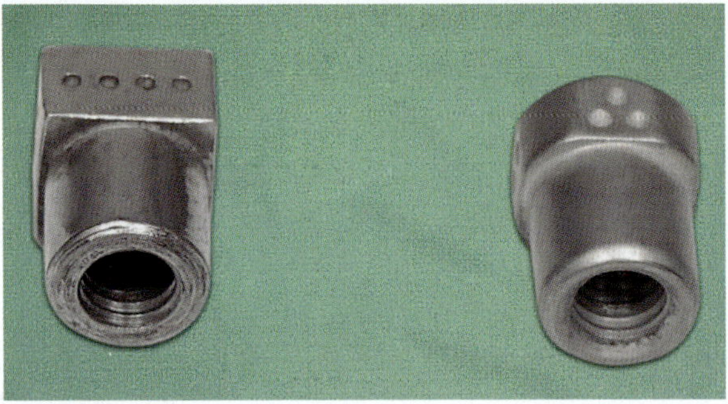

Fig. 7.16: Square head nut.

Washer

Washer is used to fill the space; these are of various types:

- Spacing washer size—1.5, 2.0 mm **(Fig. 7.17)**
- Flat-sided washer size—2.0 mm **(Fig. 7.17)**
- Slotted washer size—4.0 mm **(Fig. 7.17)**

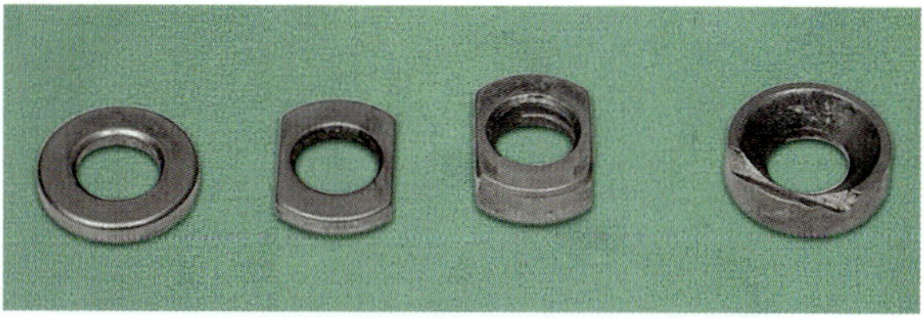

Fig. 7.17: Spacing washers, flat washers, and slotted washers.

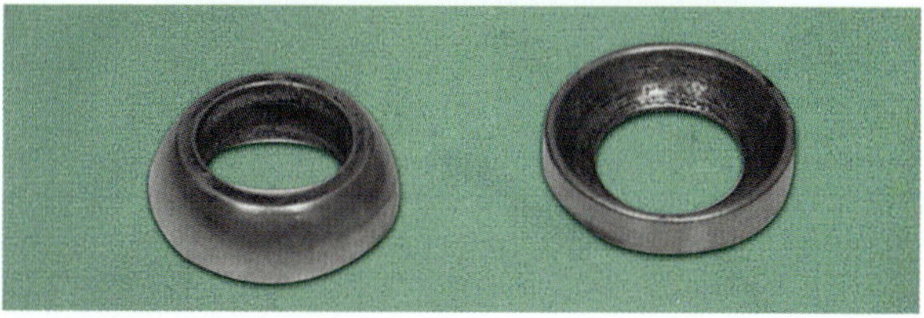

Fig. 7.18: Conical washers.

Conical Washer Couple

Conical washer couple is shown in **Figure 7.18**.

Wire Fixation Bolt

Wire fixation bolt is used to secure the wires and can be either cannulated or slotted. These are of 6 mm threaded diameter, 18 mm length, and a bolt head thickness of 6 mm. The bolt heads are either hexagonal or with two flat and rounded surfaces. Cannulated bolts have a 2 mm hole while slotted bolts have an oblique groove on the underface of the bolt head. The bolt head being double in thickness to that of a regular bolt head, it facilitates turning when the adjacent holes are occupied by other nuts/bolts **(Fig. 7.19)**.

A special cannulated bolt is also available with a head thickness of 11 mm. It has a 6 mm diameter threaded hole

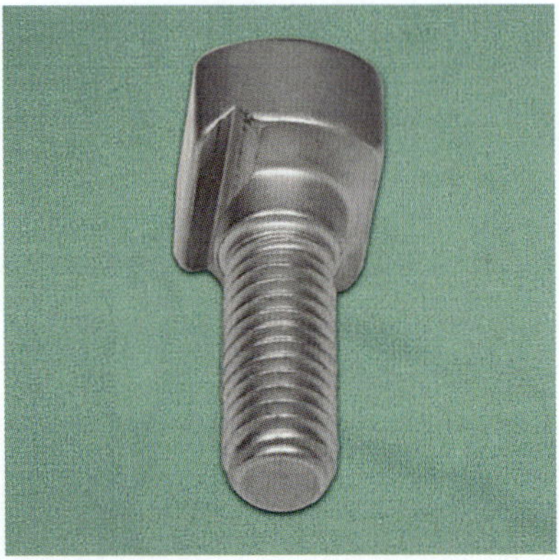

Fig. 7.19: Wire fixation bolt.

at the center of the head top, which allows introduction of bolts/rods when needed under special circumstances.

Wire Fixation Cannulated Bolt

Cannulated bolts are preferred for 1.5 mm wires and slotted bolts for 1.8 mm wires. For optimal tightening, it is advisable to use 5 mm nuts with wire fixation bolts. Because of metal fatigue, wire fixation bolts should never be reused **(Fig. 7.20)**.

Wire Fixation Bolt with Threaded Socket

The wire fixation bolt with threaded socket has dual function **(Fig. 7.21)** for fixation of wire and connecting threaded rod.

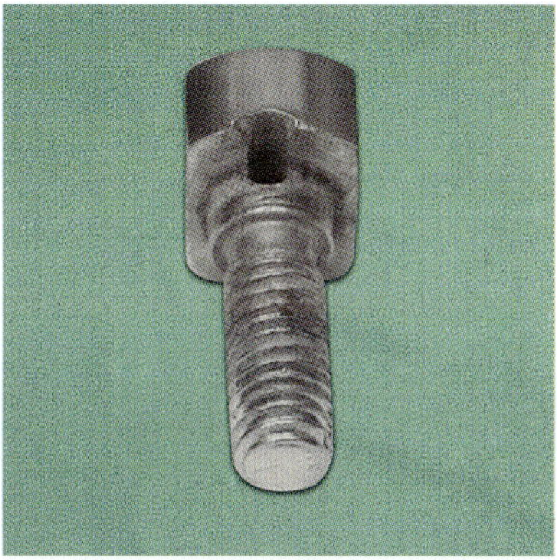

Fig. 7.20: Wire fixation cannulated bolt.

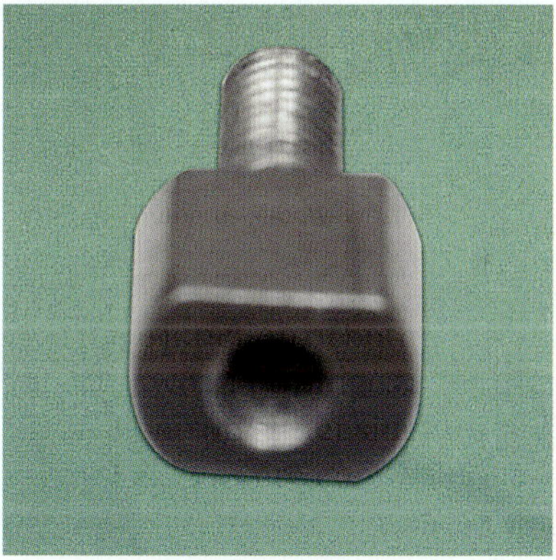

Fig. 7.21: Wire fixation bolt with threaded socket.

Block for Half Pin/Rancho Cubes

Block for half pin is shown in **Figure 7.22**.

Block for Half Pin for Center Sleeve

Block for half pin for center sleeve is shown in **Figure 7.23**.

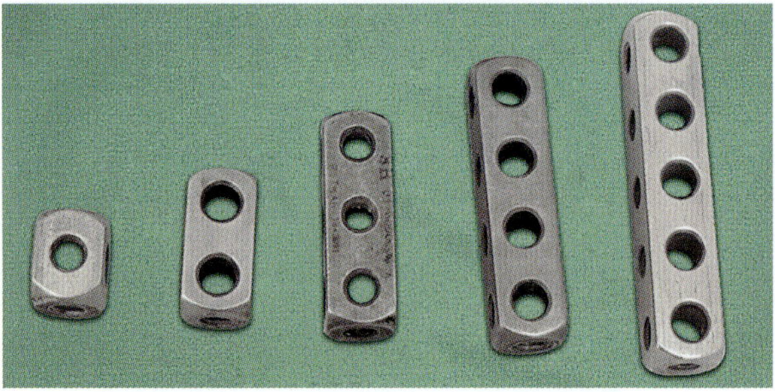

Size 1, 2, 3, 4, and 5 holes

Fig. 7.22: Block for half pin.

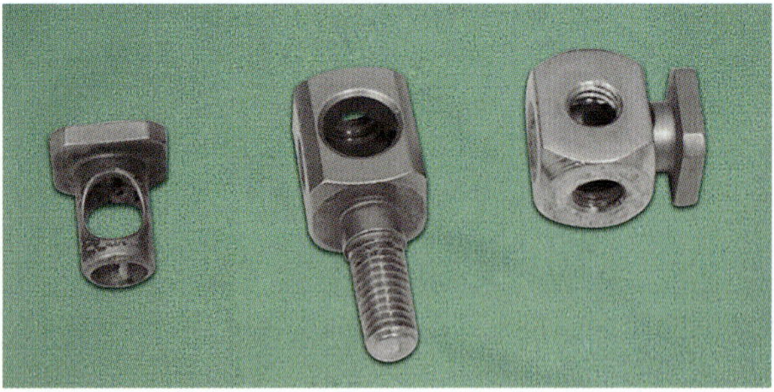

Fig. 7.23: Block with center sleeve.

Box Wrench for Bolt

Box wrench for bolt is shown in **Figure 7.24**. Box wrench is used to tight and loosen the nut.

Socket Wrench for Wire Fixation Bolt

Socket wrench is shown in **Figure 7.25**.

Combination Wrench (10 mm)

Wrench is shown in **Figure 7.26**.

Osteotome and Key

Osteotome and key are shown in **Figure 7.27**.

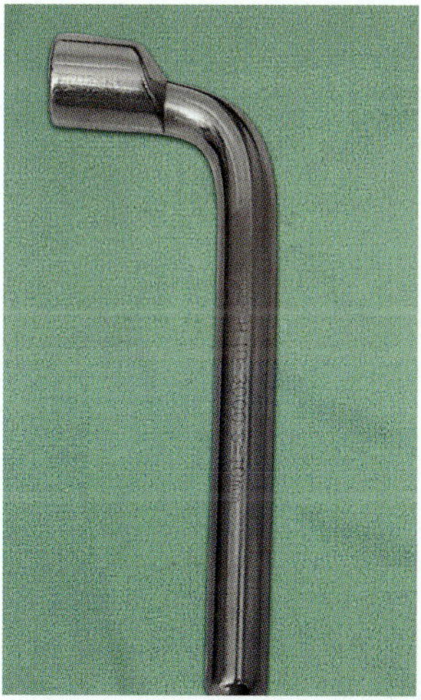

Fig. 7.24: Box wrench.

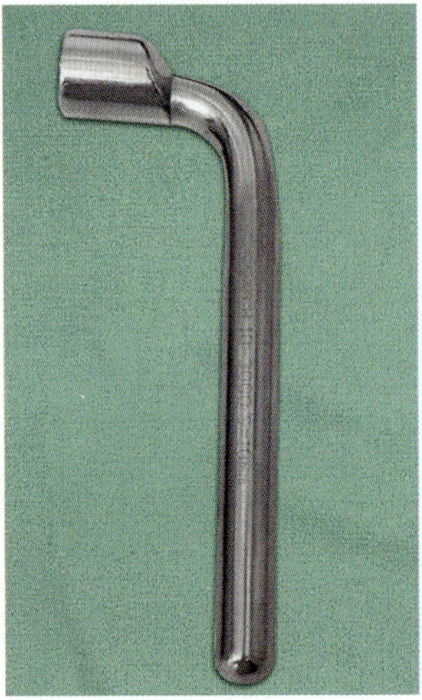

Fig. 7.25: Socket wrench.

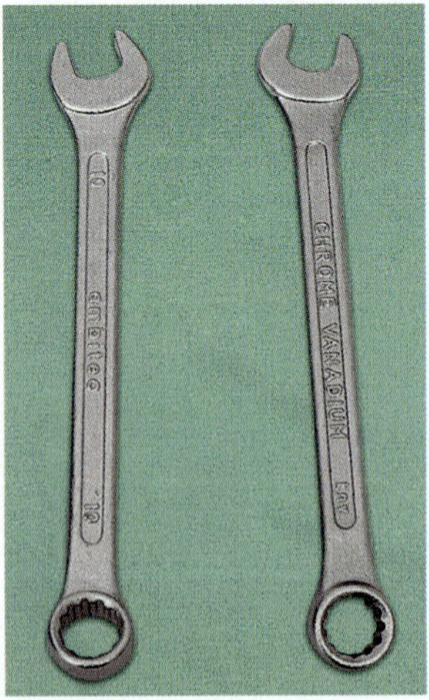

Fig. 7.26: Wrench.

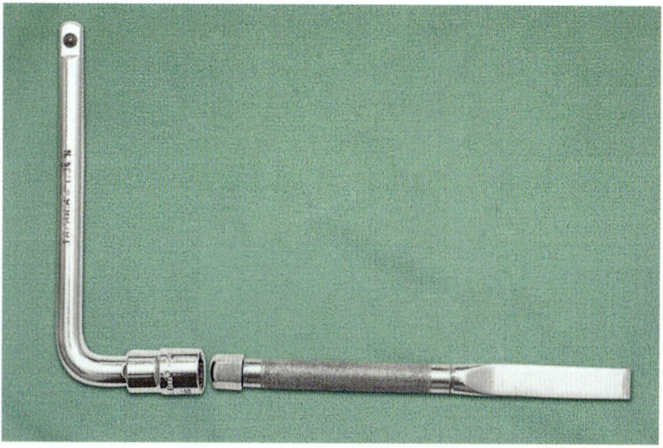

Size 3, 5, 7, and 9 mm

Fig. 7.27: Osteotome and key.

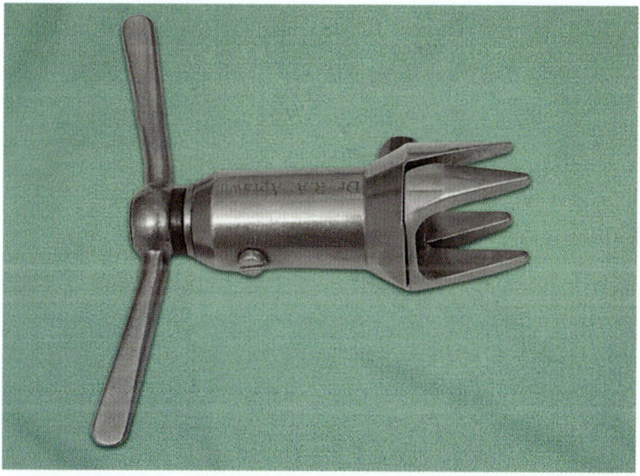

Fig. 7.28: Wire tensioner.

Wire Tensioner—Mechanical

Wire tensioner is shown in **Figure 7.28**.

Wire Tensioner Direct Measuring

Direct measuring wire tensioner is shown in **Figure 7.29**.

Corticotome

Corticotome is shown in **Figure 7.30**.

Implants

Wires:

The bayonet point ***(Fig. 7.31A)***: It is used mainly for diaphysis of long bones as it has greater penetrating power. The advantage of bayonet point is that it causes less heating effect of bones and soft tissues. It produces hole of

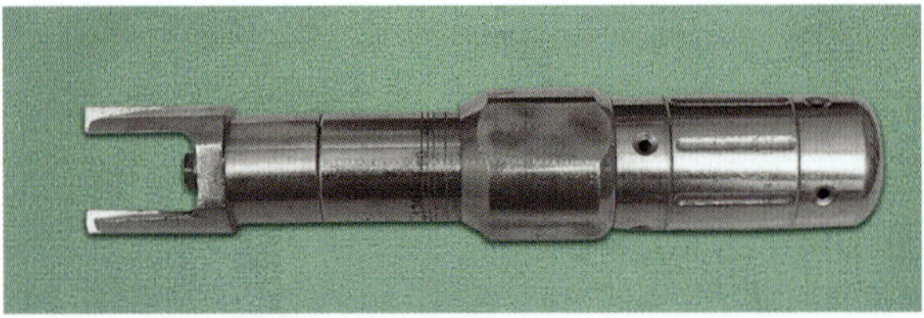

Fig. 7.29: Wire tensioner direct measuring.

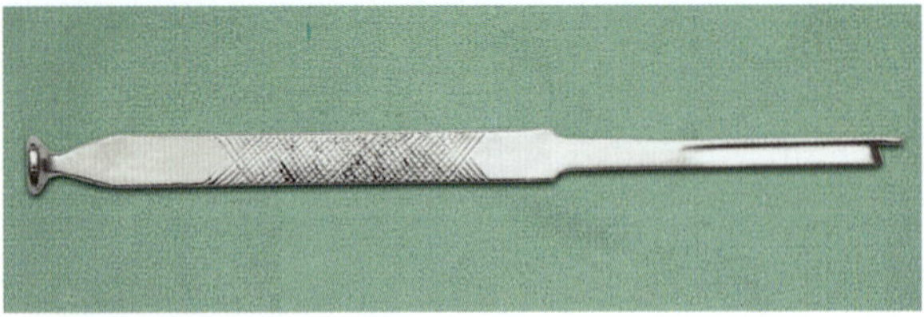

Size 3, 5, 7, and 9 mm

Fig. 7.30: Corticotome.

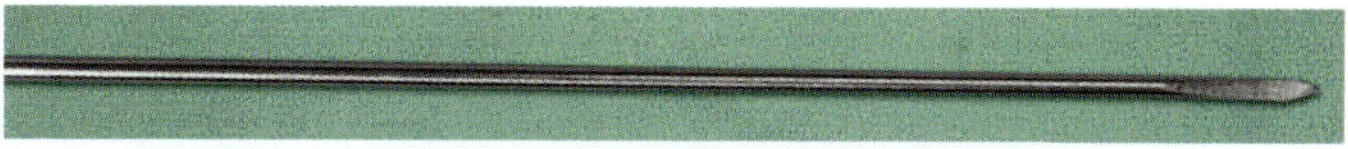

Fig. 7.31A: Bayonet point.

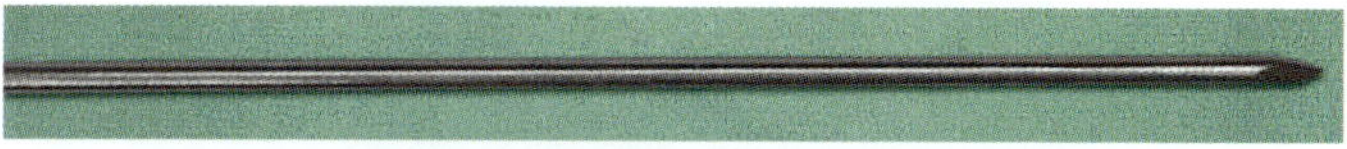

Fig. 7.31B: Trocar point.

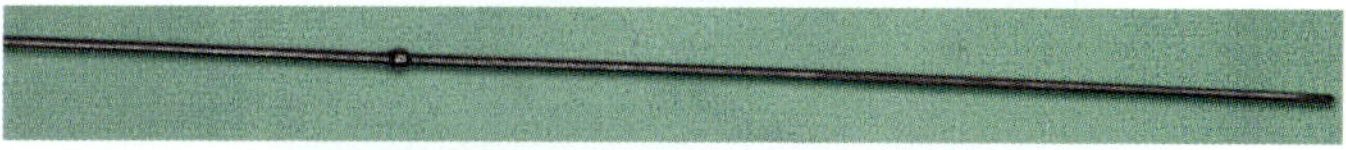

Fig. 7.31C: Olive or stopper wire.

a diameter slightly larger than that of wire thus causing less friction.

The trocar point ***(Fig. 7.31B)****:* Trocar point is used in the metaepiphyseal regions of bones because it has less penetrating power. It produces the hole of exactly the same diameter as of the wire. The advantage of trocar point is that it has greater hold in the bones.

Olive or stopper wire ***(Fig. 7.31C)****:* The olive wire is used to achieve and maintain the position of principle fragment after fracture. It is also used to hold the fragment during correction of deformities.

Ilizarov Box for Hardware

Ilizarov box for hardware is shown in **Figure 7.32**.

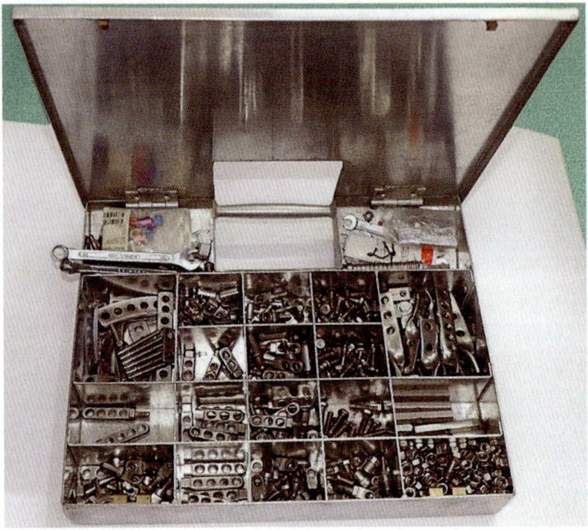

Fig. 7.32: Ilizarov box.

CHAPTER

8 Surgical Technique

SURGICAL TECHNIQUE OF CORRECTION OF CUBITUS VARUS DEFORMITY BY ILIZAROV APPARATUS

Cubitus deformity is the most common and late complication of supracondylar fractures. Many reports have been described with various osteotomy techniques to correct this three-dimensional deformity.

However, the timing of surgery, selection of osteotomy technique, and type of internal fixation to be used remain controversial.

The lateral closed wedge osteotomy is the most widely used method to correct this deformity. Despite the method's ability to restore carrying angle and preserve elbow motion, some authors have reported poor cosmetic appearance of the elbow because of lateral condylar prominence. Everybody claims their method to be the best, but high complication rates of the osteotomies have been reported in the literature.

When to do the surgery?

Surgery should be done only after allowing for maximum remodeling of the fracture. A rough estimate will be around a year after the original injury. However, patient demands, growth potential, and status of the physis should be taken into account while planning surgery.

What surgeries are available?

Most authors recommend surgery in the form of corrective osteotomies to achieve a normal carrying angle. At times, in cases with physeal arrest in young child, epiphysiodesis is needed. Various types of osteotomies have been described each claiming improvements in cosmesis as well as lesser complication rates with their techniques. The osteotomies described are lateral close wedge osteotomy, modified French osteotomy, equal limbs lateral closed wedge osteotomy, step cut osteotomy, dome osteotomy, medial open wedge osteotomy, lateral oblique osteotomy, and distraction osteogenesis. Many variations of these main techniques are reported in literature, but essential principles remain the same. The first osteotomy described by Siris was simple lateral closed wedged osteotomy which was modified by French to have intact periosteal hinge and fixation with screws and tension looped steel wires.

Principles of Surgical Technique

Cubitus varus deformity is corrected by supracondylar osteotomy. There are various methods of supracondylar osteotomy such as lateral closed wedge osteotomy, open wedge osteotomy, and other osteotomies. The basic principles of all the osteotomies are to correct the deformity. The deformity can be corrected acutely or gradually. The surgical procedures can be either open surgery or percutaneous. There are various methods of fixation, either internal or external. The methods of fixation are ranged from plate fixation, Kirschner wire fixation, screw fixation and only with plaster immobilization and external fixation that ranges from simple uniplanar fixator to Ilizarov ring fixators. The osteotomy is performed in the thinnest part of supracondylar region in both coronal plane and sagittal plane **(Fig. 8.1)**. In open surgery, the deformity is corrected immediately, whatever preferred method of internal fixation is applied. Since the bone stock is very less, there are more chances of instability of fragment. Ilizarov technique corrects the deformity gradually and the frame is quite stable. Thus, the gradual deformity correction and fixation by Ilizarov fixator is the most preferred technique.

Ilizarov Distraction Osteogenesis Technique

The Ilizarov distraction osteogenesis has several advantages in deformity surgery, such as providing adjustable, three-dimensional correction, stable fixation, and allowing immediate range of motion (ROM) with less soft tissue damage and scar formation.

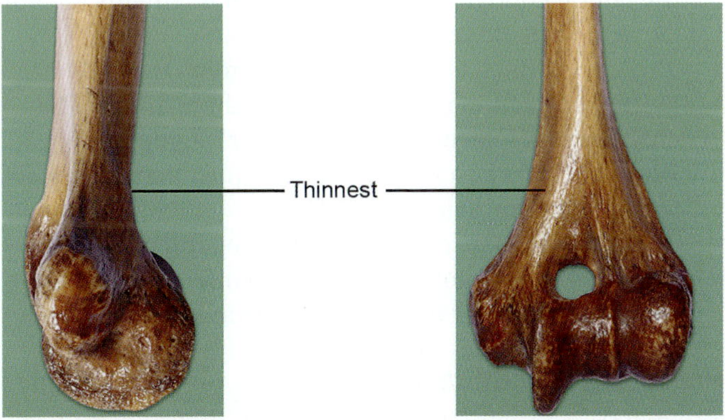

Fig. 8.1: Osteotomy site.

Principles of surgical techniques:

- In some of the cases where both varus deformity and age of the patient is less, immediate correction of total deformity is done but if the age is more and the deformity is more, the deformity is corrected gradually.
- The gradual correction of the deformity by distraction osteogenesis gives good regeneration and good callus formation.
- There are juxta-articular hinges which cause medial translation of the lower fragment during correction of the deformity.
- After correction of the varus deformity (usually after 2 weeks when the good callus is formed), internal rotation deformity is corrected by derotation of the fragment.
- The Ilizarov fixator is very versatile and deformity correction is under control.
- Since no open surgery is done thus, periosteum is not disturbed.
- In the close wedge deformity, the lateral prominence of the lateral condyle is avoided as both fragments are not close to each other.
- The lazy S, which is a common deformity, is avoided.
- During correction of the deformity, there are minimum chances of displacement of the lower fragment.
- Physiotherapy is started next day, thus, the stiffness of the joint is eliminated.
- There are very less chances of the deep infection.
- There are chances of minor pin tract infection which can be eliminated after removal of the fixator.

Preconstructed Frame

Two full rings of appropriate size are selected. The diameter of the ring must be two finger larger than the limb being operated upon at the maximum diameter. The distal ring is positioned at the level of the epicondyles, above this level is olecranon fossa and coronoid fossa, this wires and half pins can be applied without damaging the olecranon fossa. If the wires or half pins passed through the olecranon fossa, the movement at the elbow joint may be restricted. Proximal ring is placed at the anterior axillary fold. The ring cannot be placed below the axillary fold because at this level the radial nerve is passing. The wires and half pins can damage the radial nerve. Both rings are connected by threaded rods and juxta-articular hinges. This juxta-articular hinges are placed in the sagittal plane anteriorly and posteriorly on the distal ring. The tilting of distal ring is calculated by total amount of correction needed, i.e., summing up the amount of varus deformity and humerus–elbow–wrist (HEW) angle of the normal side.

The first olive wire is inserted from posterolateral aspect of the lateral epicondyle to the anterior cortex of the medial epicondyle at 6–8° valgus inclination to the joint lines **(Fig. 8.2)**.

Preconstructed frame is attached to the first olive wire **(Fig. 8.3)**.

Second olive wire is passed at the proximal ring from anterolateral to posteromedial direction **(Fig. 8.4)**.

Tensioning of the first olive wire is done at the distal ring **(Fig. 8.5)**.

Tensioning of the second olive wire is done at the proximal ring **(Fig. 8.6)**.

Third olive wire is inserted from medial epicondyle, direction posteromedial to anterolateral, ulnar nerve is protected by palpating and pushing it away from the point of insertion of wire **(Fig. 8.7)**.

Tensioning of the third olive wire is done **(Fig. 8.8)**.

Drilling by 2.5 mm drill bit through a protective sleeve for half pin at lateral condyle, direction posterolateral to anteromedial **(Fig. 8.9)**.

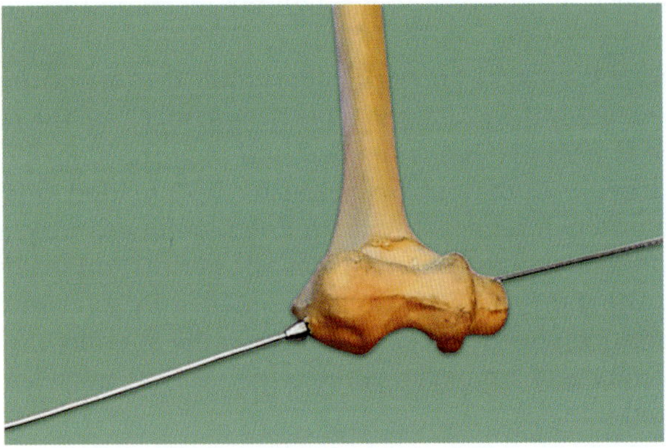

Fig. 8.2: Olive wire is passed from posterolateral to anteromedial surface.

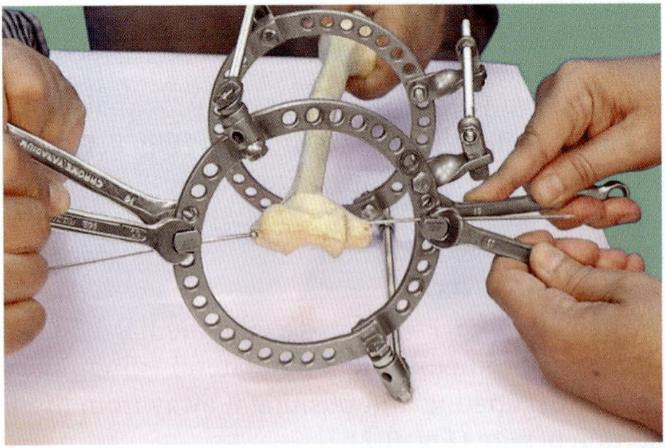

Fig. 8.3: Preconstructed frame is attached tightening the first olive wire.

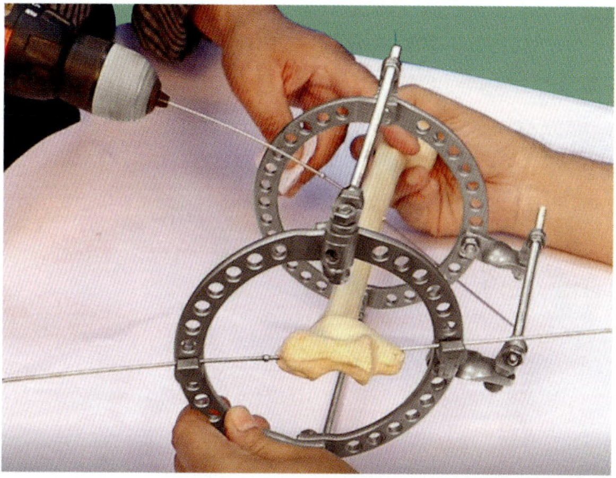

Fig. 8.4: Proximal ring is at the level of the anterior axillary fold and wire is passed from anterolateral to posteromedial.

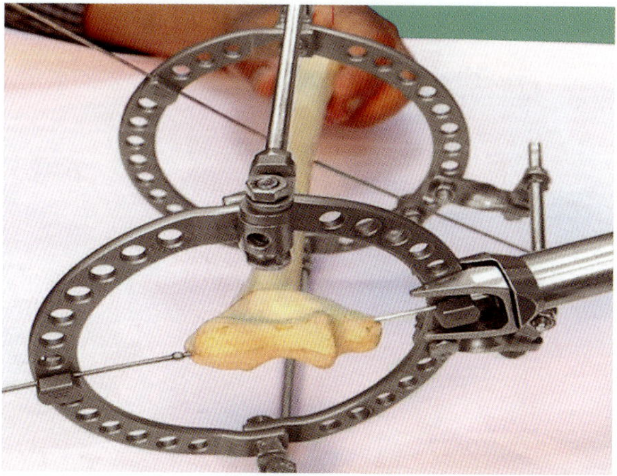

Fig. 8.5: Tensioning of first olive wire.

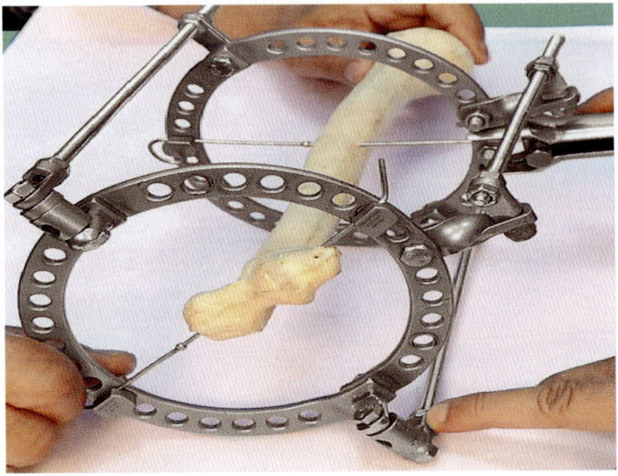

Fig. 8.6: Tensioning of the second wire.

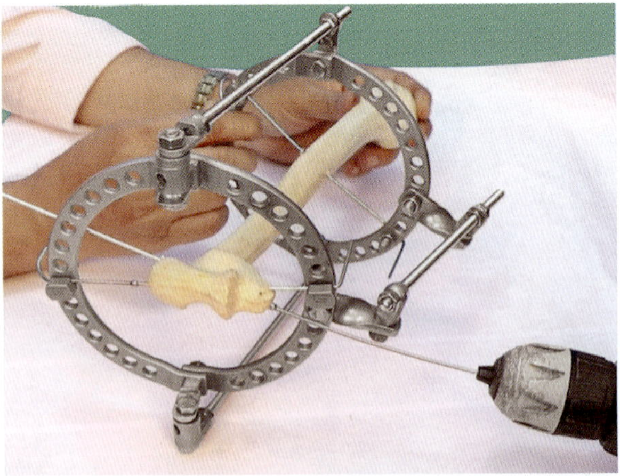

Fig. 8.7: Insertion of third wire from medial epicondyle, direction posteromedial to anterolateral, ulnar nerve is protected.

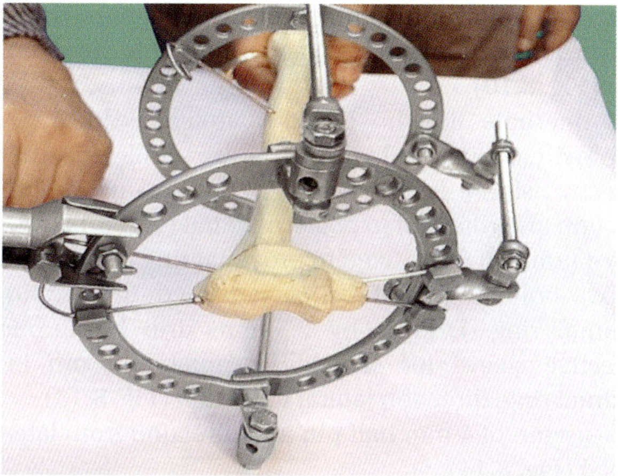

Fig. 8.8: Tensioning of third wire.

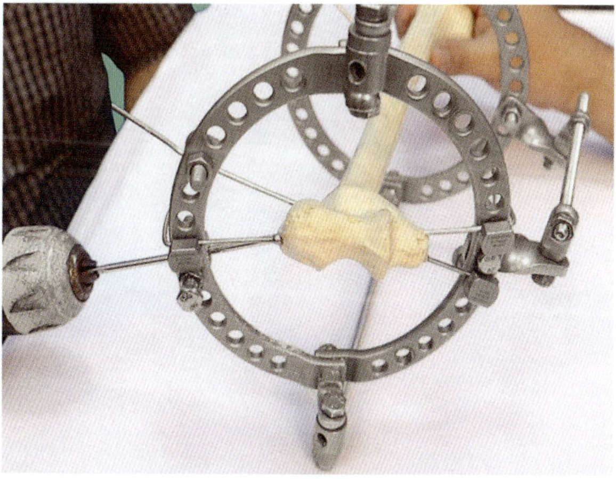

Fig. 8.9: Drilling by 2.5 mm drill bit for half pin in the distal ring at lateral condyle, direction posterolateral to anteromedial.

A 4 mm half pin is inserted to strengthen the distal fixation, taking care to avoid placement within the olecranon fossa **(Fig. 8.10)**.

A one-hole Rancho block is attached downward to the proximal ring. Drilling by 2.5 mm drill bit through a protective sleeve for the distal half pin at proximal ring, direction anterolateral to posteromedial **(Fig. 8.11)**.

A 4 mm half pin is fixed to proximal ring **(Fig. 8.12)**.

Two-hole Rancho block is attached upward to the proximal ring. Drilling by 2.5 mm drill bit through a protective sleeve for second proximal half pin in the proximal ring, direction lateral to medial **(Fig. 8.13)**.

Insertion of 4 mm half pin and direction from lateral to medial **(Fig. 8.14)**.

The final positioning of the frame is confirmed under C-arm.

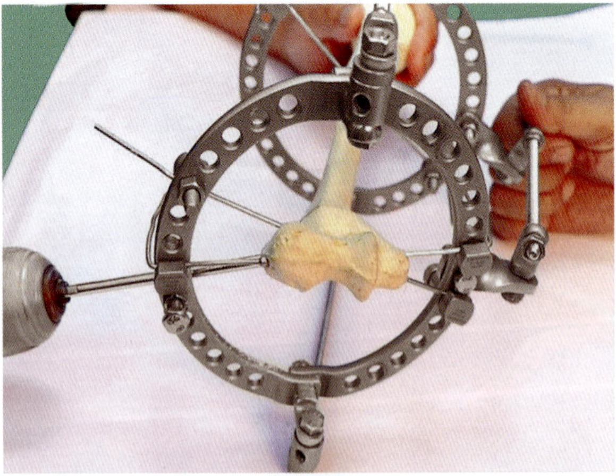

Fig. 8.10: Insertion of 4 mm half pin at lateral condyle, direction posterolateral to anteromedial.

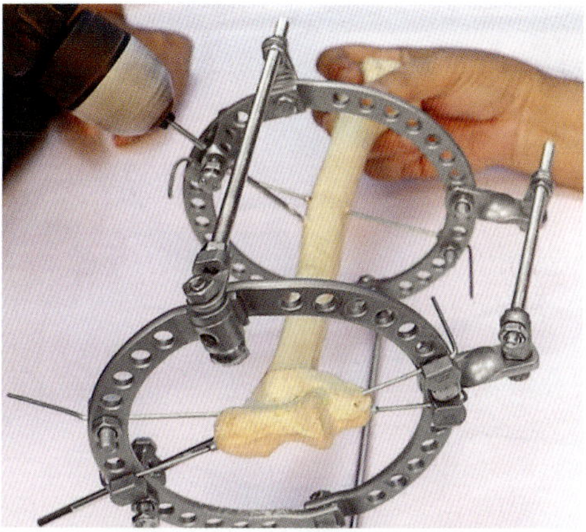

Fig. 8.11: One-hole Rancho block is attached downward to the proximal ring. Drilling by 2.5 mm drill bit through a protective sleeve for the distal half pin at proximal ring, direction anterolateral to posteromedial.

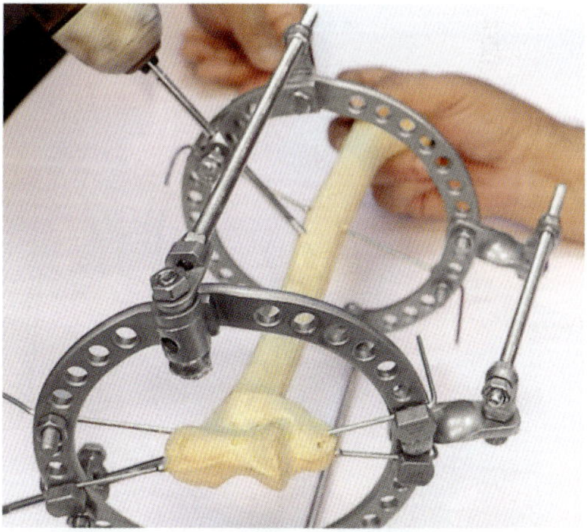

Fig. 8.12: A 4 mm half pin is fixed to proximal ring, direction anterolateral to posteromedial.

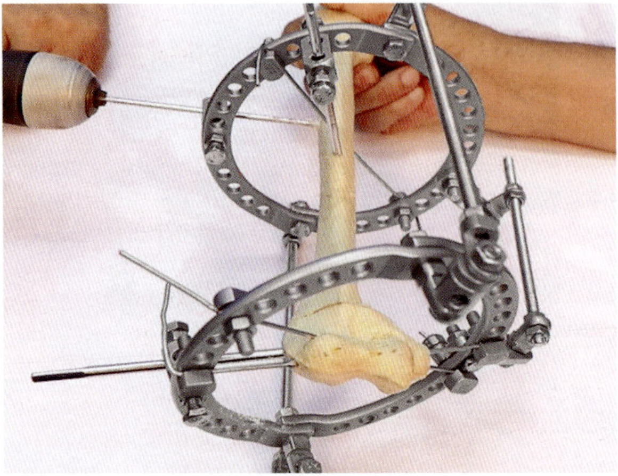

Fig. 8.13: Two-hole Rancho block is attached upward to the proximal ring. Drilling by 2.5 mm drill bit through a protective sleeve for second proximal half pin in the proximal ring, direction lateral to medial.

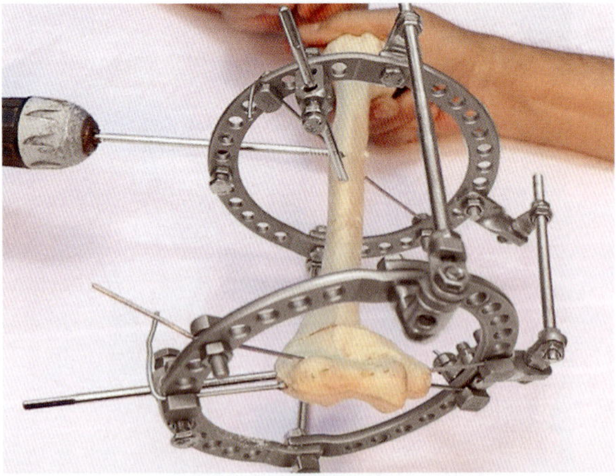

Fig. 8.14: Insertion of 4 mm half pin, direction lateral to medial.

The level of osteotomy is above the olecranon fossa and the level of the osteotomy confirmed under C-arm.

A 1.5–2 cm sized stab incision up to periosteum was made along the lateral supracondylar ridge. Subperiosteal dissection is performed at the osteotomy site.

Loosening of anterior hinge and posterior hinge before osteotomy to get space for the osteotomy **(Figs. 8.15 and 8.16)**.

Preosteotomy drilling by 2.5 mm drill bit, direction from lateral to medial, anterolateral to posteromedial, and posterolateral to anteromedial **(Figs. 8.17 to 8.19)**.

Supracondylar osteotomy is performed by osteotome, direction from lateral to medial **(Fig. 8.20)**.

Surgical Techniques

Clinical measurements and radiographs (AP and lateral) of both elbows were reviewed preoperatively and the amount

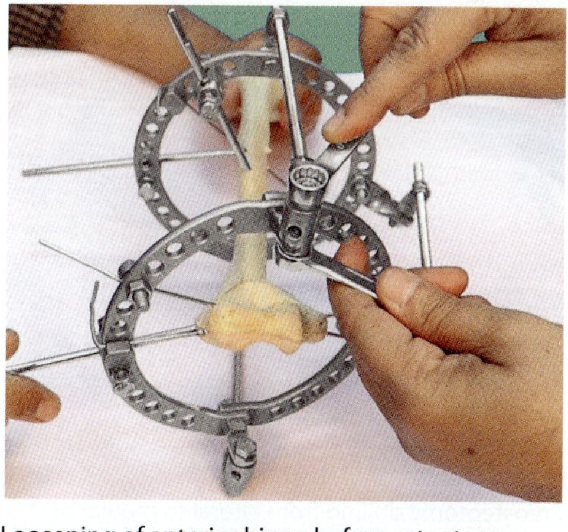

Fig. 8.15: Loosening of anterior hinge before osteotomy.

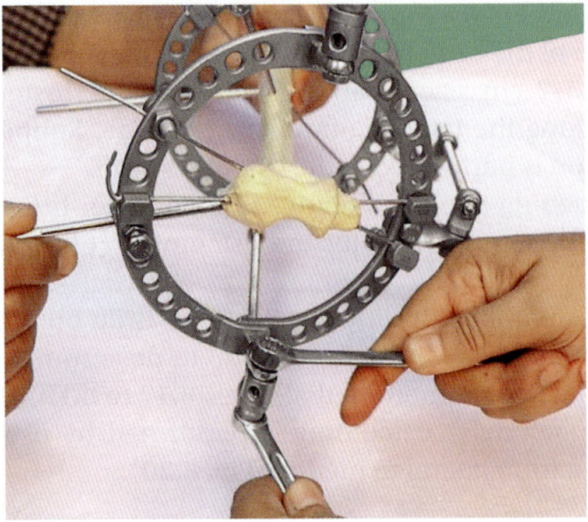

Fig. 8.16: Loosening of posterior hinge.

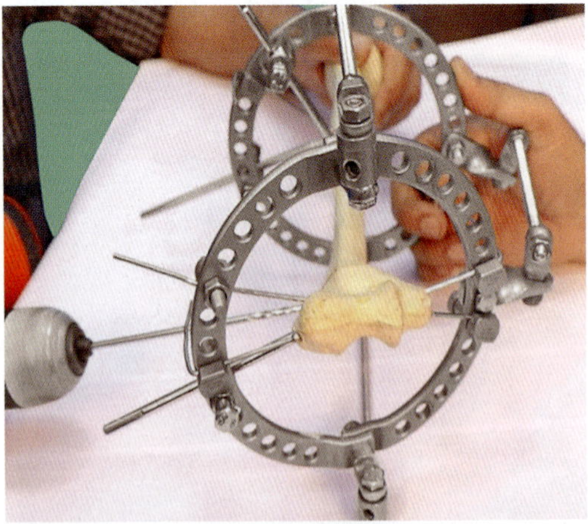

Fig. 8.17: Preosteotomy drilling from lateral to medial by 2.5 mm drill bit.

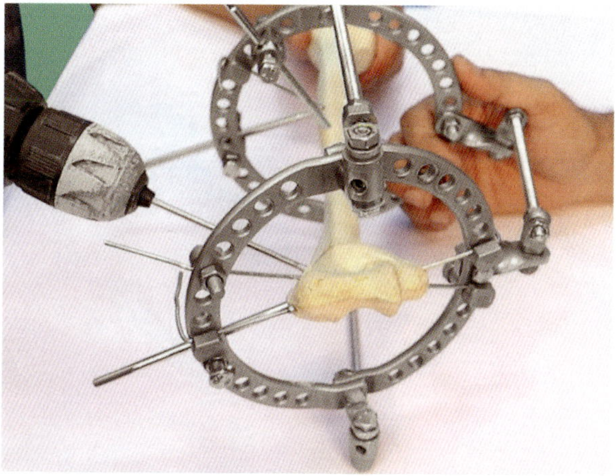

Fig. 8.18: Drilling for osteotomy, direction anterolateral to posteromedial.

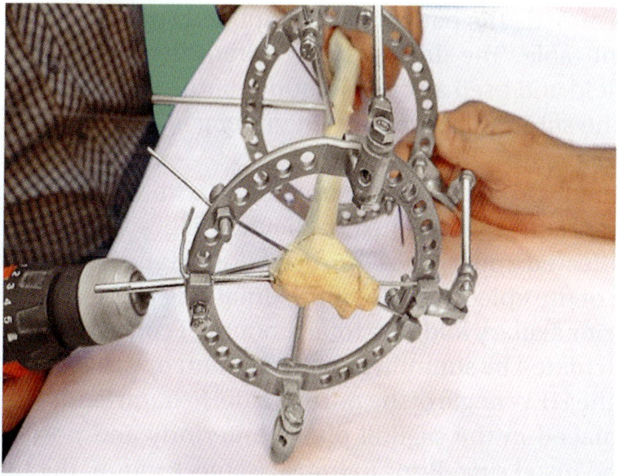

Fig. 8.19: Drilling from posterolateral to anteromedial.

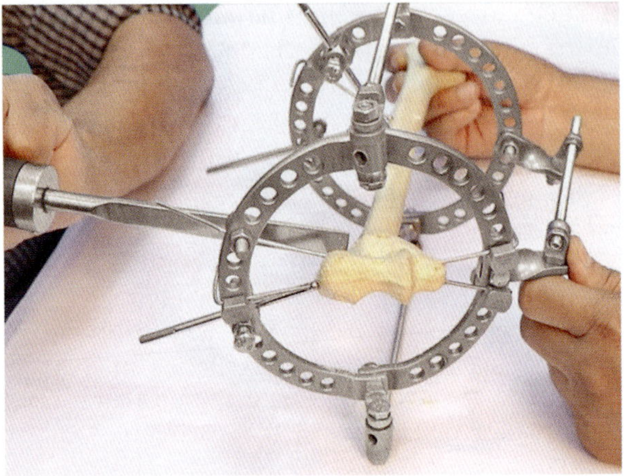

Fig. 8.20: Supracondylar osteotomy, direction lateral to medial cutting anterior and posterior cortex.

of surgical correction required to achieve symmetry was determined. The patient was positioned supine on a radiolucent table. The draped image intensifier is focused into the field and used as the operating stand.

The surgery was performed under general anesthesia or brachial plexus block.

The preconstructed Ilizarov frame with two full rings of appropriate sizes and juxta-articular hinges is mounted on the affected upper limb. The distal ring was positioned at the level of the epicondyles and proximal ring at the level of the anterior axillary fold. The total amount of correction needed is calculated by summing up the amount of varus deformity and the HEW angle of the normal side. Juxta-articular hinges are placed in the sagittal plane, anteriorly and posteriorly on the distal ring. Prior to transosseous fixation, the hinges were loosened and the distal ring was positioned 6–8° of valgus inclination to the joint line under C-arm guidance. The distraction assembly is affixed perpendicular to the hinge axis on the medial side of the arm.

The first olive wire is inserted from posterolateral aspect of the lateral epicondyle to the anterior cortex of the medial epicondyle at 6–8° valgus inclination to the joint lines taking care to avoid placement within the olecranon fossa.

Preconstructed frame is attached to the first olive wire **(Fig. 8.21)**.

Second olive wire is passed at the proximal ring from anterolateral to posteromedial direction.

Tensioning of the first olive wire is done at the distal ring.

Tensioning of the second olive wire is done at the proximal ring **(Fig. 8.22)**.

Third olive wire is inserted from medial epicondyle, direction posteromedial to anterolateral, ulnar nerve is protected by palpating and pushing it away from the point

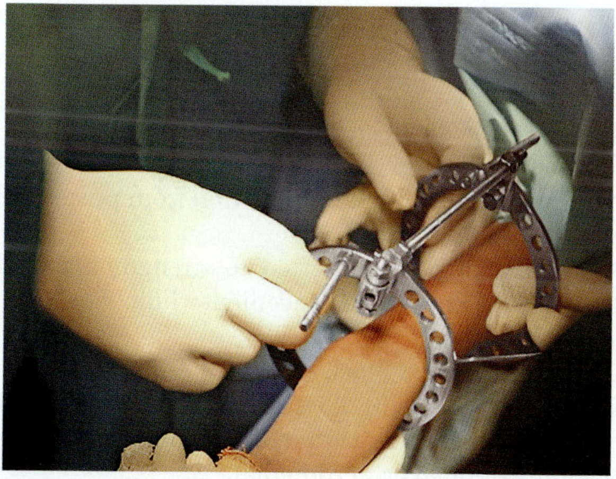

Fig. 8.21: Preconstructed frame.

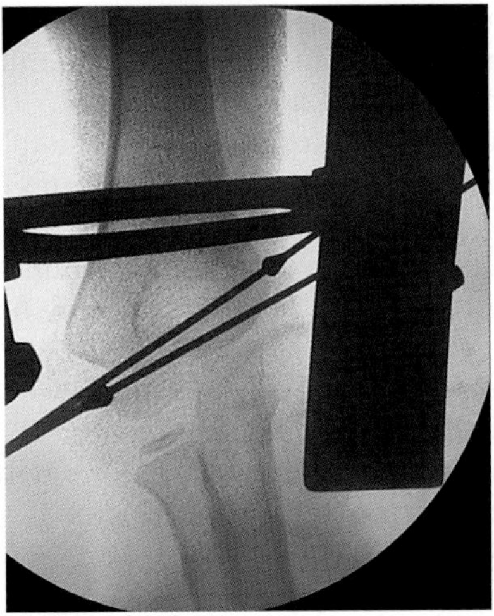

Fig. 8.22: The olive wires in the lateral epicondyle and the medial epicondyle are passed taking care to avoid placement within the olecranon fossa.

of insertion of wire taking care to avoid placement within the olecranon fossa.

Tensioning of the third olive wire is done.

Drilling by 2.5 mm drill bit through a protective sleeve for half pin at lateral condyle, direction from posterolateral to anteromedial.

A 4 mm half pin is inserted to strengthen the distal fixation, taking care to avoid placement within the olecranon fossa.

One-hole Rancho block is attached downward to the proximal ring. Drilling by 2.5 mm drill bit through a protective sleeve for the distal half pin at proximal ring, direction from anterolateral to posteromedial.

A 4 mm half pin is fixed to proximal ring.

Two-hole Rancho block is attached upward to the proximal ring. Drilling by 2.5 mm drill bit through a protective sleeve for second proximal half pin in the proximal ring, direction from lateral to medial.

Insertion of 4 mm half pin, direction from lateral to medial.

The final positioning of the frame is confirmed under C-arm.

The level of osteotomy is above the olecranon fossa and the level is confirmed under C-arm.

The lateral supracondylar ridge is palpated **(Fig. 8.23)**.

A 1.5–2 cm sized stab incision up to periosteum was made along the lateral supracondylar ridge. Subperiosteal dissection is performed at the osteotomy site.

Loosening of anterior hinge and posterior hinge before osteotomy to get space for the osteotomy.

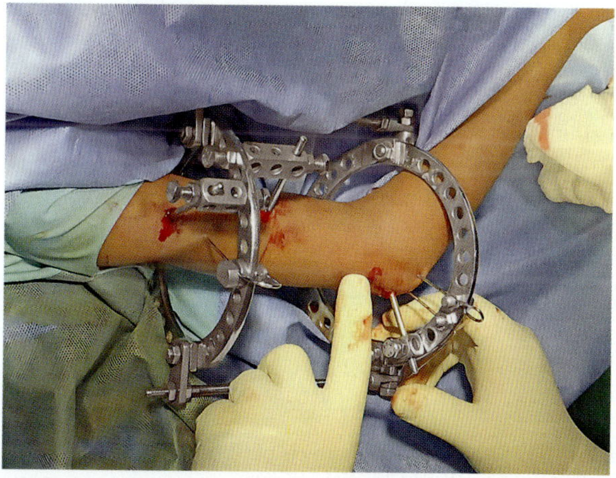

Fig. 8.23: Lateral supracondylar ridge is palpated.

Preosteotomy drilling by 2.5 mm drill bit, direction from lateral to medial, anterolateral to posteromedial, and posterolateral to anteromedial.

Supracondylar osteotomy is performed by osteotome, direction from lateral to medial **(Fig. 8.24)**.

Gradually the deformity is corrected by distracting the motor unit on medial side, there is translation of the lower fragment on the lower side due to juxta-articular hinges (principles of osteotomy Rule 2) **(Figs. 8.25 and 8.26)**.

After correction, both rings become parallel and four threaded rods are applied. Anterior and posterior hinges with threaded rods are removed. All the threaded rods are tightened.

X-ray to be done to visualize good callus formation **(Figs. 8.27 to 8.29)**.

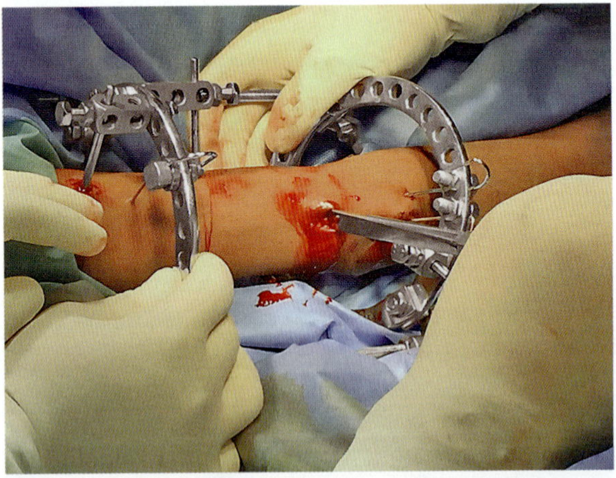

Fig. 8.24: Supracondylar osteotomy is performed.

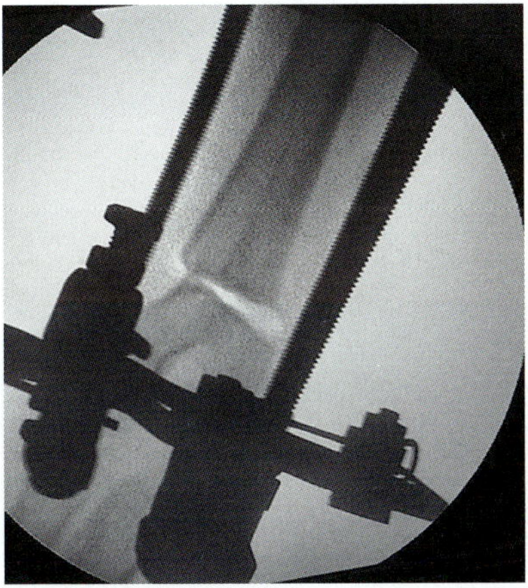

Fig. 8.25: The lower fragment is translated medially during correction due to juxta-articular hinges.

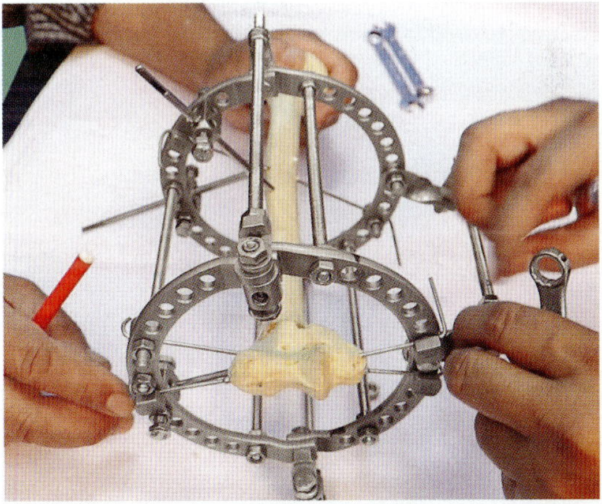

Fig. 8.26: Lateral condyle prominence is avoided by compensatory medial translation of the lower fragment of the humerus (Dror Paley Osteotomy Rule 2).

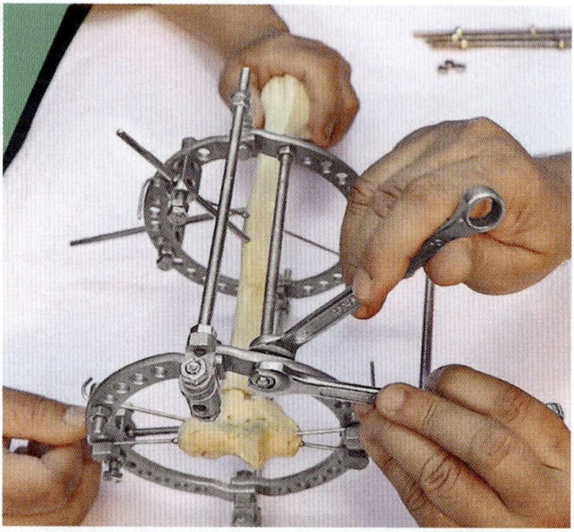

Fig. 8.27: After correcting varus deformity, two more threaded rods are added to make the frame stable.

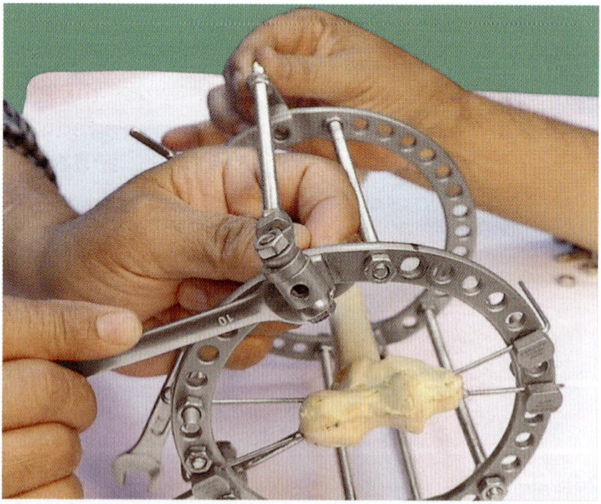

Fig. 8.28: Anterior and posterior hinges are tightened.

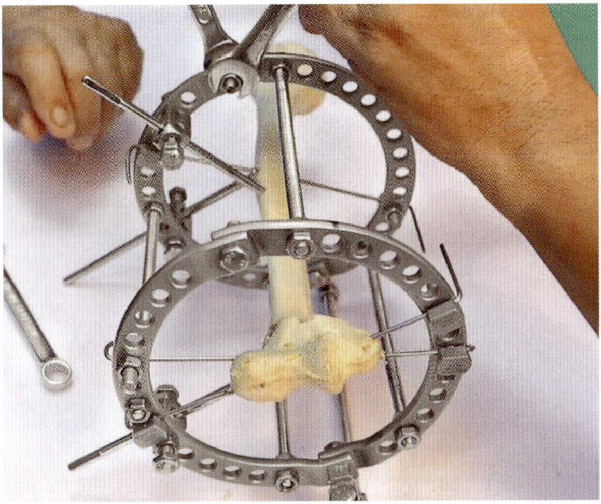

Fig. 8.29: Cubitus varus deformity is corrected.

To correct internal rotation of the distal humerus, the fragment was derotated 10° by shifting all the threaded rods of the distal ring by one hole in the desired direction during the postoperative period **(Figs. 8.30 and 8.31)**. This maneuver was performed only after some callus formation occurred at the osteotomy site, i.e., at an interval of 2–3 weeks following the primary surgery.

Figures 8.32 and 8.33 show construction of frame and incision for osteotomy.

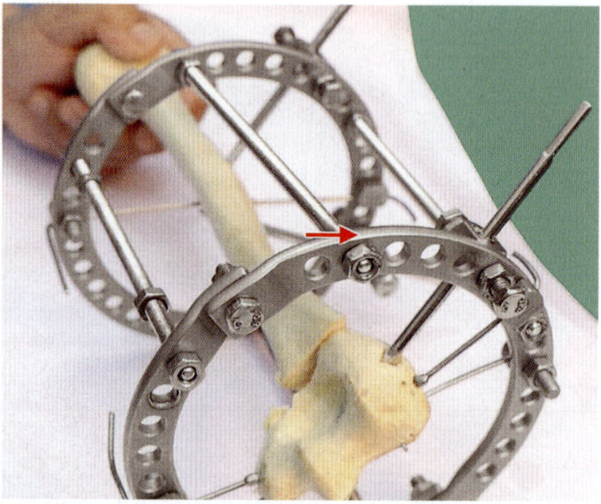

Fig. 8.30: To correct internal rotation of distal humerus, the fragment is derotated by 10° shifting all the threaded rods one hole clockwise in the distal ring.

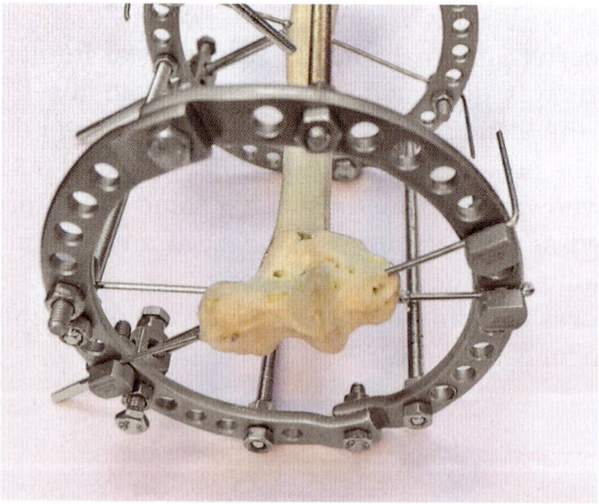

Fig. 8.31: Threaded rods are tightened resulting in 10° derotation of the distal fragment.

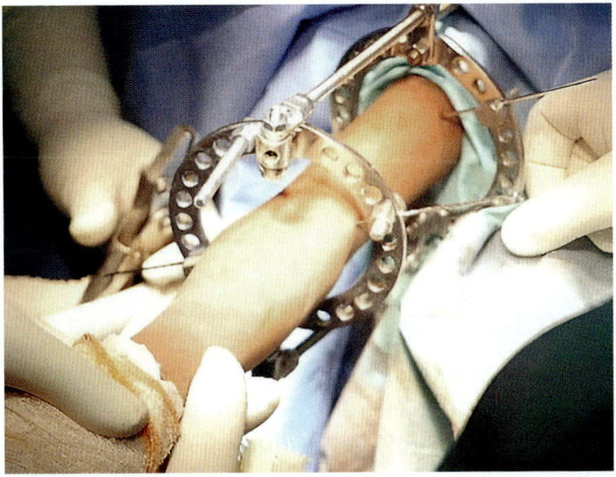

Fig. 8.32: Preosteotomy frame.

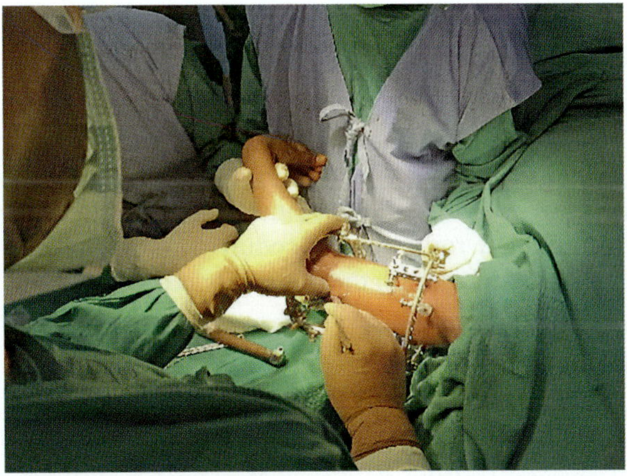

Fig. 8.33: Incision for osteotomy.

CHAPTER

9 Postoperative Management

INTRODUCTION

Postoperative pin tract and wound should be taken care. Elbow and shoulder exercises are initiated as soon as the pain subsides. Basically, in the elbow flexion and extension, supination and pronation exercises are started. The varus deformity is corrected by gradual distraction motor unit on medial side starting from day 7 four times a day. The rate of distraction is calculated by the rule of similar triangles.

DISTRACTION TECHNIQUE

Motor unit rod is distracted at proximal male hinge by turning the nut exactly one-fourth of the full turn. The opposite nut is loosened. One-fourth turn (90°) causes 0.25 mm distraction. After this, the first nut must be tightened firmly at the threaded rod. This procedure is adopted at 7 AM, 11 AM, 3 PM, and 7 PM till the deformity is corrected.

RULE OF SIMILAR TRIANGLES (FIG. 9.1)

A mid-diaphyseal line is drawn at the proximal fragment of the humerus, and a mid-diaphyseal line is drawn at the distal fragment of the humerus. Proximal and distal lines are connected to each other, the intersection of these lines

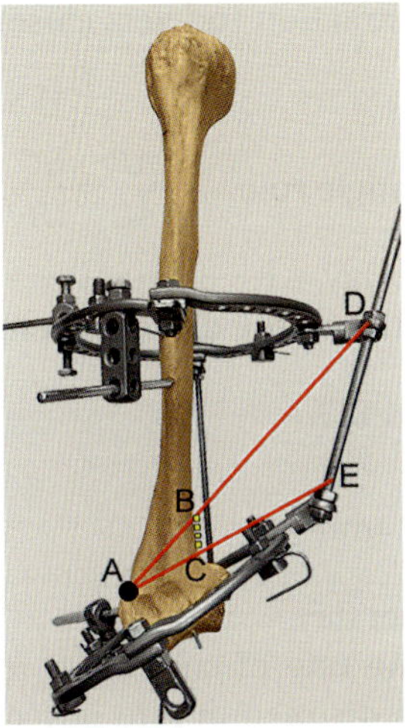

Fig. 9.1: Before correction.

is called as CORA. The angle formed by the two axes at the CORA is a measure of angular deformity in that plane. The line joining the concave angulated cortex of the bone and CORA is extended on the convex cortex of the bone. The deformity will be distracted from the convex cortex of the bone, assuming a distraction rate of 1 mm per day at the concave cortex of the bone (BC). We want to know the rate of distraction at the distraction rod (DE). This can be expressed as follows—if BC = 1 mm, how much will DE be? This can be calculated as a simple ratio of AD to AB compared with DE to 1, where AD is the perpendicular distance from the hinge to the distraction rod and AB is the shortest distance from the hinge to the concave cortex. Because the correction is being performed in a circular fashion around the hinge, the rate may need to be recalculated intermittently, as the distance of the distraction rod gets closer to the bone with time.

Example:

The similar triangle rule: → $\frac{AB}{AD} = \frac{BC}{DE}$

BC = 1 mm per day, AB = 3 cm, AD = 9 cm, then

Rate of distraction at the distraction rod

$$(\text{DE}) = \left(\frac{AD}{AB}\right) \times \text{BC}$$

$$= \left(\frac{9}{3}\right) \times 1 \text{ mm}$$

$$= 3 \text{ mm per day.}$$

To calculate the rate of correction for distraction of a hinge, assuming a distraction rate of 1 mm per day at the concave cortex of the bone (BC), we want to know the rate of distraction at the distraction rod (D). This can be expressed as follows—if BC = 1 mm, how much will DE bc? This can be calculated as a simple ratio of AD to AB compared with DE to 1, where AD is the perpendicular distance from the hinge to the distraction rod and AB is the shortest distance from the hinge to the concave cortex. Because the correction is being performed in a circular fashion around the hinge, the rate may need to be recalculated intermittently as the distance of the distraction rod gets closer to the bone with time.

After correction, both rings became parallel and a compensatory medial translation of distal fragment occurred due to the juxta-articular hinges **(Fig. 9.2)**.

AD (before correction) = 9 cm

AD (during distraction) = 6 cm

So, the rate of correction will be changed from 3 mm per day to 2 mm per day.

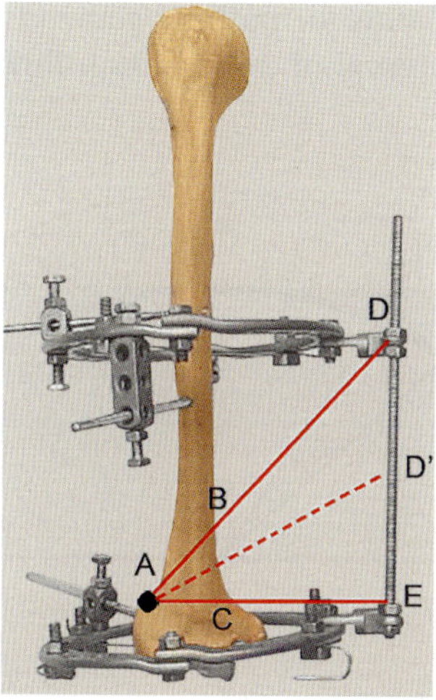

Fig. 9.2: After correction.

Derotation is done to correct the internal rotation deformity. For it, borders and the holes of the selected ring is traced on a paper and then angle (x) subtended by two adjacent holes is calculated **(Figs. 9.3A and B)**. The number of holes (n) is calculated by dividing the total internal rotation deformity (y) and angle between two adjacent holes (x), i.e., n = is the number of holes through which derotation has to be done to achieve maximum possible correction and avoid overcorrection of internal rotation deformity **(Fig. 9.4)**. To correct internal rotation of the distal humerus, the fragment is derotated by shifting all the threaded rods of the distal ring by one hole in the clockwise direction. All the threaded rods are tightened, producing anticlockwise movement of the distal ring and the distal humeral fragment is rotated externally **(Fig. 9.5)**. This maneuver is performed only after some callus formation occurred at the osteotomy site, i.e., at an interval of 2–3 weeks following the primary surgery.

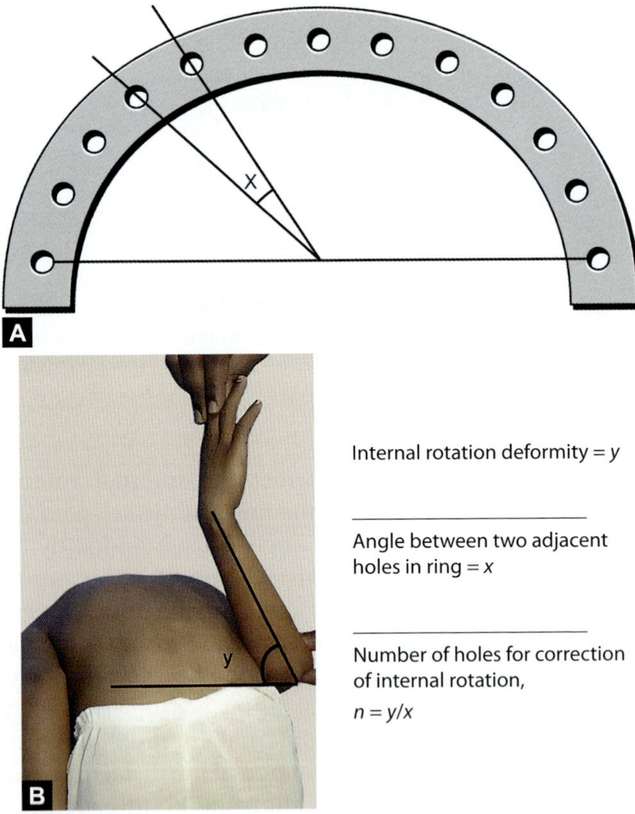

Figs. 9.3A and B: A tracing of the outer and inner borders and holes of the ring selected for deformity correction. x is the angle between two adjacent holes. y is the internal rotation deformity measured by Yamamoto method.

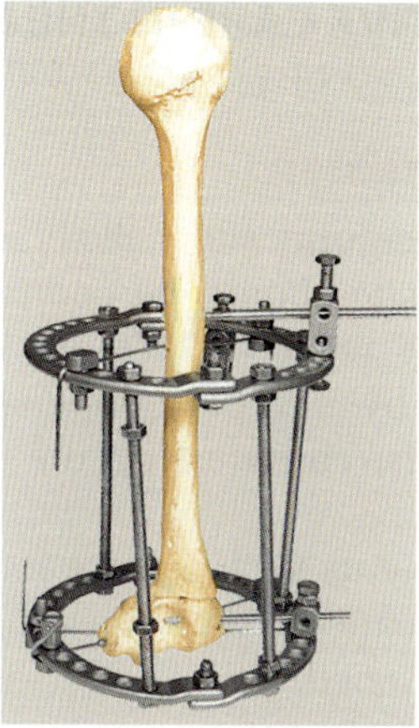

Fig. 9.4: To correct internal rotation of distal humerus, the fragment is derotated by shifting all the threaded rods one hole clockwise in the distal ring.

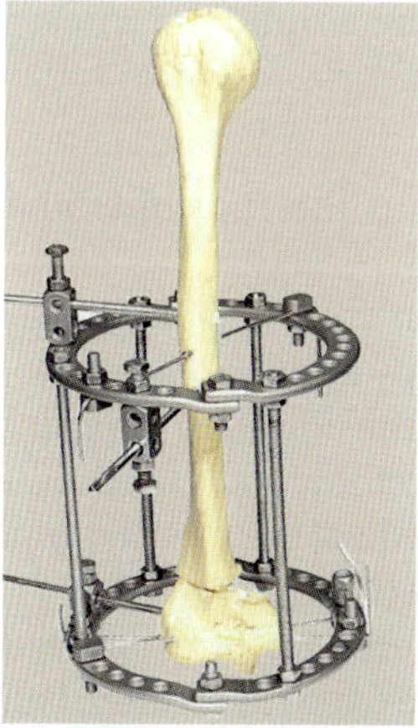

Fig. 9.5: Threaded rods are tightened proximally and distally. The ring is rotated anticlockwise resulting external rotation of lower humeral fragment.

POSTOPERATIVE CARE IN THE ILIZAROV METHOD

In Operation Theater

Sometimes the osteotomy site is likely to bleed, to prevent it, the osteotomy site should be compressed. There may be bleeding at the wires or half pin sites, the bleeding can be prevented by external tamponade in the form of large dressing pads, compressing the skin around these areas.

All the components such as wire fixation bolt, Rancho at the half pins, threaded rods, hinges, nuts, and bolts in the frame must be tightened.

The wires cut and bent smoothly, and half pin cut as short as possible with the cut ends covered by tape.

Check range of movements (ROMs) of the elbow joint, if there is any restriction by any wire or half pin, surgical release must be done around the wires.

Pain Relief

- Pain control in the postoperative period is most important.
- If adequate pain control is done, patient will cooperate for physiotherapy and mobilization.
- Pain will cause the adoption of protective postures, such as flexion of the elbow leads to elbow flexion contracture.
- Contracture is one of the most common "complications" of the Ilizarov technique.
- Pain after surgery can be produced by overstretching acute correction of the deformity. Pain can be relieved by loosening the threaded rods or sometimes by loosening of wires.

- Next day in the ward, the care should be taken for any loosened wire fixation bolt, Rancho attached to half pin, nut and bolts at the hinges and threaded rods.

Limb Positioning

- Proper limb positioning minimizes the chances of development of contractures.
- There is a tendency to keep the elbow in flexion; instruct the patient to keep his elbow in extension.

The Distraction Phase

The threaded rods are marked with tape. Distance moved on the threaded rod of motor unit has to be compared regularly for proper distraction. It is also confirmed lethargically.

Range of Movements of Adjacent Joints

Early active and passive ROM of the elbow is started as soon as possible. Full ROM of shoulder and wrist encouraged. Occasionally, frame may need to be modified to allow full flexion (cut the anterior portion of distal ring) **(Fig. 9.6)**.

Neurological Examination

During follow-up check, the ulnar nerve and radial nerve for motor and sensory function to be checked. In the ulnar nerve injury, there is numbness and tingling at the middle and little finger. The wire passing at the medial epicondyle close to the ulnar nerve should be loosened. If the numbness and tingling are not improved, wire should be removed. In case the radial nerve is damaged, the wires and half pins at the proximal ring which are close to radial nerve should be removed. If the damage is noticed only after the

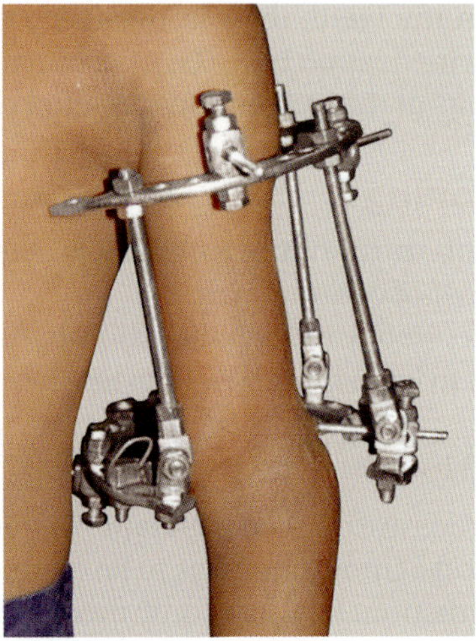

Fig. 9.6: 2/3 ring allows full flexion.

motor weakness has occurred, the chances of recovery are diminished. The usual sequence of events in neurological injury during distraction is hyperesthesia, anesthesia, and motor weakness.

Pin Sites for Signs of Inflammation/Infection

Pin sites should be cleaned with sterile saline or antiseptic lotion. Gauze dressings around the pins and wires should be changed regularly. If there is any redness and pain around a pin site associated with increased or purulent discharge, the patient can go for antibiotics.

Stability of Frame and Components

During follow-up, check-up is made to ensure that the various bolts and nuts are adequately tighten. If any instability is found, then the loose nuts should be tightened immediately.

Follow-up (X-rays)

In sequential X-rays, measure the humerus–elbow–wrist (HEW) angle. At the end of distraction, HEW angle of both limbs should be same.

Quality of the Regenerate

Initially, there is shadowy streaks of linear ossification by the end of 3 weeks. This ossification should show progressive improvement over subsequent X-ray examinations.

Physiotherapy

The patient has to participate in a proper program of physiotherapy and mobilization. In lack of proper physiotherapy, even the technically excellent surgery yields poor result.

The Consolidation Phase

At the end of distraction, Ilizarov recommends *"Training the Regenerate"*. During the consolidation phase, encourage the full elbow ROMs.

Removal of the Fixator and Postfixator Removal

"A month too late is better than a day too early." Fixator removal is done after clinical and radiological union which was determined by the presence of bridging callus across the osteotomy site in 3 out of 4 cortices in two orthogonal views. Clinical assessment of union is performed by loosening the connecting rods between the two rings and testing for mobility in two planes. Actual removal of the fixator is usually done under anesthesia. In adults, though it is possible to do without anesthesia, but it is not recommended, as the removal of half pins is quite painful. In case a removal is done without anesthesia, one must remember to loosen the wire fixation bolts, thus releasing wire tension prior cutting of wires. When the last wire is cut, ensure that the limb does not drop suddenly. Remember to inject local anesthetic at the site of the olive, when removing olive wires. Use of braces or casts is usually not necessary.

CHAPTER

10 Errors and Complications

PROMINENT LATERAL CONDYLE

Usually for correction of cubitus varus, the osteotomies are performed at supracondylar region, above the level of olecranon fossa. If the lower humeral fragment is translated laterally, prominent lateral condyle deformity occurs. We have used juxta-articular hinges, osteotomy rule 2 for correction of the cubitus varus deformity, which leads to medial translation of lower humeral fragment. In spite of juxta-articular hinges, if hinges are not properly loosened to get space at the osteotomy site and if the direction of osteotomy is not in the bisector line, the lower humeral fragment may be translated laterally, instead of medial translation and produces the lateral condyle prominence **(Figs. 10.1 to 10.3)**.

PIN TRACT INFECTIONS

Pin tract infection is the most common complication in Ilizarov technique. Prevention of pin tract infection by continuous irrigation while drilling the wires and pins prevents the heat necrosis. Drilling should be done by low rpm speed, and always be intermittent instead of continuous drilling.

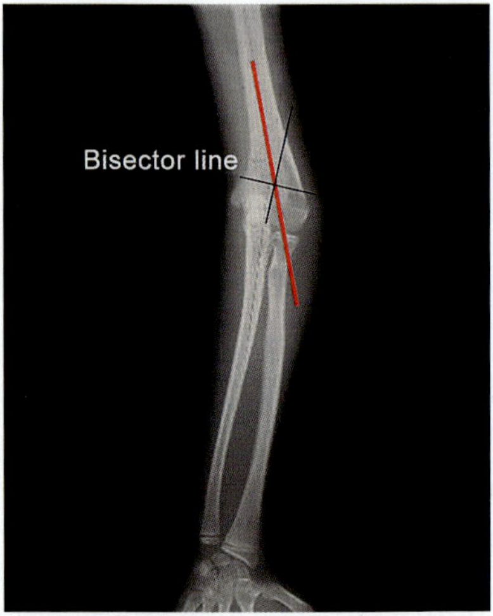

Fig. 10.1: X-ray showing cubitus varus deformity.

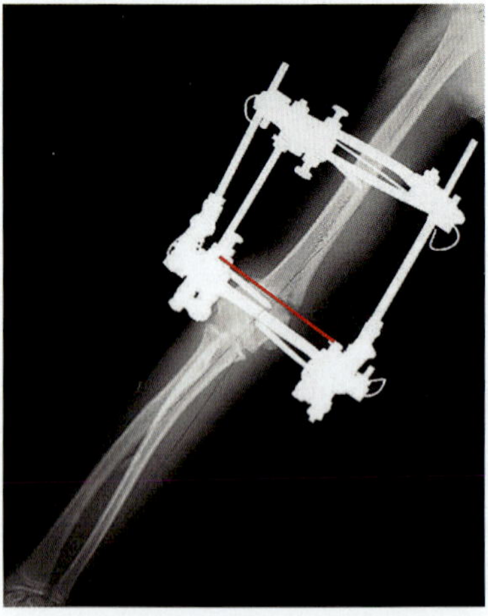

Fig. 10.2: The direction of osteotomy is transverse not in bisector line.

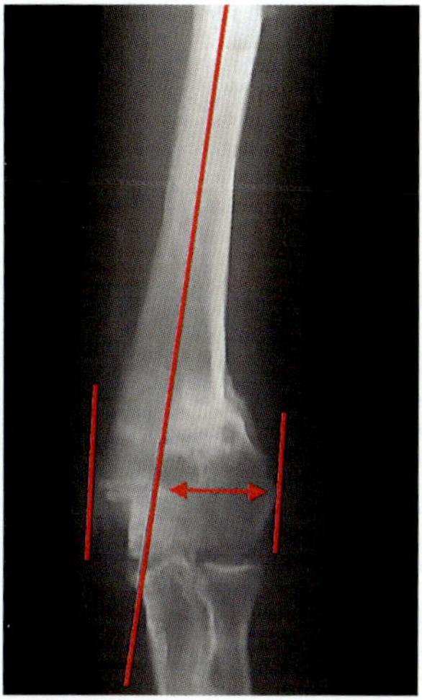

Fig. 10.3: In spite of medial translation of humerus-elbow-wrist angle, there is lateral translation.

Pin tract infection is treated by regular antiseptic dressing and oral antibiotics, rarely necessitating the systemic antibiotics. If pin tract infection persists in spite of regular antiseptic dressing and antibiotics, we need to exchange the pin. Usually pin tract infection subsides after removal of pin.

ULNAR NERVE INJURY

Ulnar nerve can be damaged while inserting the wire from the medial epicondyle. Ulnar nerve should always be protected by palpating the nerve and pushing it away from the wire insertion point.

PROTECTION OF THE OLECRANON FOSSA

The wires and pins are inserted through the medial epicondyle and lateral epicondyle. The care should be taken not to pass through the olecranon fossa.

TRACTION INJURY TO THE NERVE

If the deformity is corrected acutely, there may be chances of traction injury to the nerve. This can be avoided by acute correction of the deformity which is not more than 10°.

UNDERCORRECTION AND OVERCORRECTION

If the pre- and postoperative planning is not done properly, it will lead to under- or overcorrection. This complication can be prevented by accurately measuring the deformity angle pre- and postoperatively, both clinically and radiologically.

NONUNION

If the speed of distraction is not regulated, it can lead to poor regeneration of callus, ultimately may go to nonunion.

REFRACTURE

If the frame is removed before solid union radiologically and clinically, there are chances of refracture.

FAILURE OF FIXATION

The frame consists of external ring which is connected to each other by threaded rods and is fixed to the bone by small diameter steel wires. These wires fasten the bone in an axial cross, through a central axis perpendicular to the plane of the bone end and they are tightened to the rings by fixation bolts to provide assembly stability. The proper operation of the device depends mainly on the wire tension, which, in turn, depends on the torque applied to the bolts that hold the wires in place. The failure of these wire fixation bolts may compromise the Ilizarov frame stability.

SHATTERING AT THE OSTEOTOMY SITE

Shattering of the fragments at the osteotomy site can happen if the predrilling before osteotomy is not done. It is advisable that the osteotomy should be performed very gradually.

RADIAL NERVE INJURY

The half pins and the wires should be inserted at the anterior axillary fold for the proximal ring. Care should be taken so that there is no damage to the radial nerve.

RECURRENCE OF DEFORMITY

The recurrence of deformity can happen, if the early removal of the frame is done before consolidation of the bone.

LOSS OF MOTION

If proper postoperative physiotherapy is not done, it can lead to the stiffness of elbow joint.

VASCULAR INJURY

The olive wire at the lateral epicondyle is passed from the posterolateral surface, the wire will be emerging at the anteromedial surface. If the wire is passed more lateral, it will damage the brachial artery and can lead to heavy bleeding.

ERRORS

- *Improper planning*: If the proper planning is not done, it can lead to many complications such as undercorrection, overcorrection, and translation of the fragments in wrong direction.
- *Error in construction of frame*: During construction of the frame, the distance between the two rings should be equal both on the anterior and the posterior side. The mechanical stability of the frame can be achieved only by three rods in-between 2 rings, placed at 120° position **(Fig. 10.4)**. The 120° position cannot be maintained due

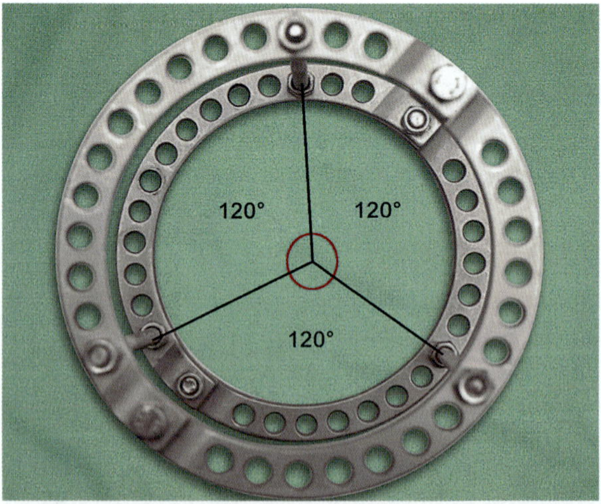

Fig. 10.4: Between two ring, three rod at position of 120° is a must.

to wire fixation bolt and junction of the ring. Thus, four threaded rods are applied.

- *Placement of the hinges*:
  - *Position of the hinges*: Both the axes of the hinge should be at the same line, any deviation from the axis will change the path of fragment motion, and it will become difficult later to control the fragments and ultimately malunion and nonunion will occur.
  - *Speed of the distraction*: The speed of the fragment should be very well regulated, so that new bone formation takes place within time, and ultimately this will not go into delayed union or nonunion.
  - *Strain on the hinges*: There should be no strain on the hinges. Sometimes, if the movements of the hinges are not proper, it produces severe pain due to crushing of the fragments.
- *Position of distraction rod*: For accurate smooth distraction, the distraction rod is always kept perpendicular to the hinges. Any deviation from the distraction rod will change the path of the movements and the rings and will lead to improper corrections.
- *Placement of wires*:
  - If the wires are not placed in the proper anatomical plane, it can lead to the damage of nerves and vessels.
  - While putting the wires, care should be taken not to obstruct the muscle movement, e.g., if the wires are placed at the posterior side, flexion movements should be checked and if the wires are from the anterior side, extension movement should be checked.
- *Placement of half pins*:
  - Proper size of the half pin is very essential, because the humerus bone is narrow in diameter.

  - The pin should be placed usually at the lateral side, to avoid damage to the nerves and vessels.
- *The level of osteotomy*: The level of osteotomy in supracondylar is very important. If the osteotomy is very close to the olecranon fossa, it will damage the olecranon fossa and if the osteotomy is away from the supracondylar region, it can damage the radial nerve.
- *Failure to calculate proper rate and rhythm*: Proper rate and rhythm are necessary to correct the deformity. The rate is decided by *"Rule of Similar Triangles"*. Any miscalculation in the rate will lead to poor regeneration and ultimately to nonunion.
- *When to stop distraction*: At the end of distraction period, upper limb alignment must be carefully evaluated, both clinically and radiologically. Any additional deformity should be corrected at this stage.
- *Removal of frame*: It is essential that the patient is carefully accessed during the consolidation period. Early removal of the frame will lead to refracture.

CHAPTER

11 Case Examples

CASE EXAMPLES

Case 1

Brief Clinical History

A young girl aged 11 having cubitus varus deformity of the left elbow. She has got fracture supracondylar at the age of eight. At that time, she was treated with casting. She complains of the pain while doing heavy work.

Preoperative Clinical Photos

- Clinically, carrying angle of the elbow is measured, while the elbow is in full extension and forearm is in supine position **(Fig. 11.1)**.
- The carrying angle of the affected elbow was 12° varus.
- The carrying angle of the normal elbow was 8° valgus.
- Clinically the total correction was 20°.

Preoperative Radiographs

- The humerus-elbow-wrist (HEW) angle of the affected elbow was 11° varus.
- The HEW angle of the normal elbow was 8° valgus.
- The total correction was 19° **(Figs. 11.2 and 11.3)**.

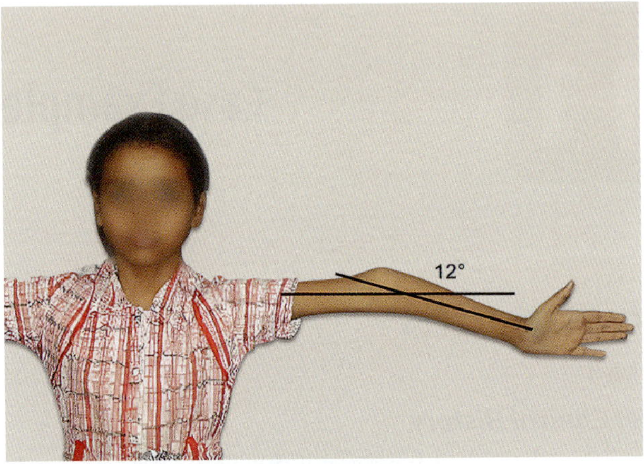

Fig. 11.1: Carrying angle of 12° of varus.

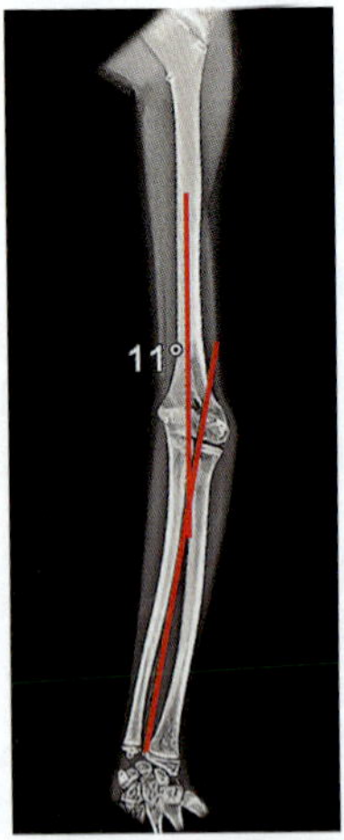

Fig. 11.2: Humerus-elbow-wrist (HEW) angle—11° varus (affected side).

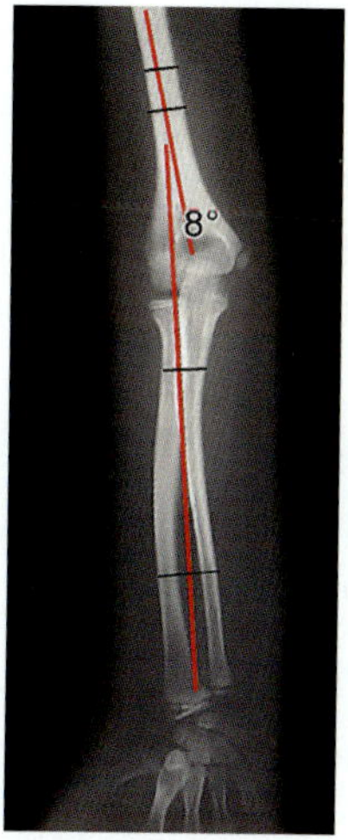

Fig. 11.3: Humerus-elbow-wrist (HEW) angle—8° valgus (normal side).

Treatment Strategies

To avoid problems with extensive scars and impaired joint movements, we decided to apply Ilizarov frame for correction of cubitus varus after supracondylar open wedge osteotomy. Preconstructed frame was prepared with two rings connected with hinges. The angulation of the distal ring was according to the total deformity corrected (20°).

The frame was fixed with the two olive wires and half pins in the distal ring and two olive wires and half pins in the proximal ring. Supracondylar osteotomy was performed. The deformity was corrected after seven days by gradual distraction by rule of similar triangles. The full correction was achieved and the both rings become parallel. The 10° internal rotation was corrected by anticlockwise derotation of the distal ring by shifting the threaded rods one hole in clockwise direction.

Postoperative Management

Proper cleaning of the wires and pins was done. Physiotherapy was started as soon as the pain subsided **(Figs. 11.4 and 11.5)**.

Removal of the Frame

Frame was removed after 10 weeks which was confirmed clinically and radiologically.

Outcome Clinical Photos and Radiographs

At final follow-up, the deformity was corrected, fully rather 2° beyond with achievement of full flexion and extension.

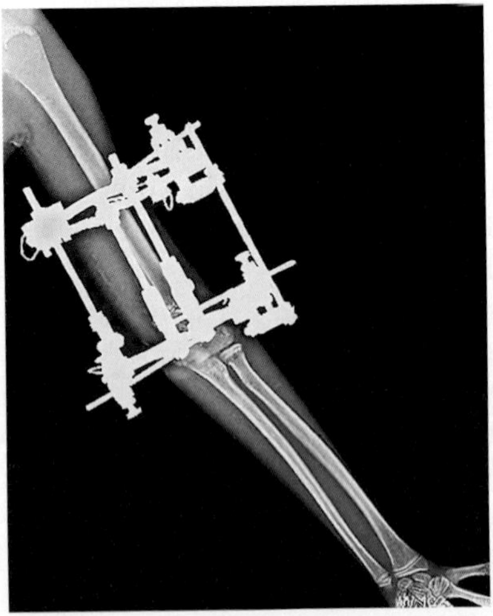

Fig. 11.4: Postoperative X-ray of elbow showing Ilizarov frame.

Radiologically, the HEW angle is 10° valgus whereas preoperative HEW angle of normal elbow was 8° valgus **(Figs. 11.6A and B and 11.7)**.

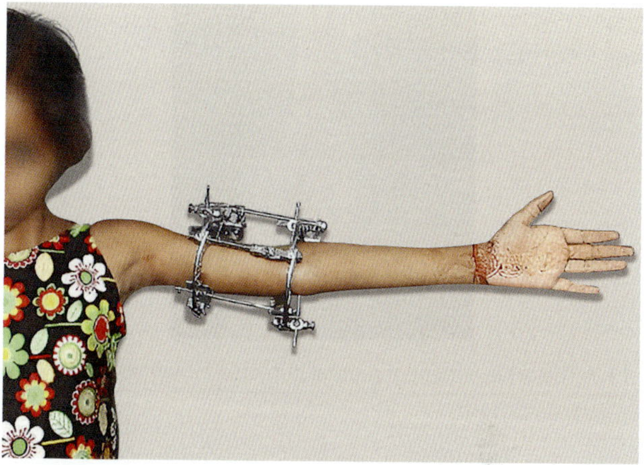

Fig. 11.5: Postoperative clinical photo with Ilizarov frame.

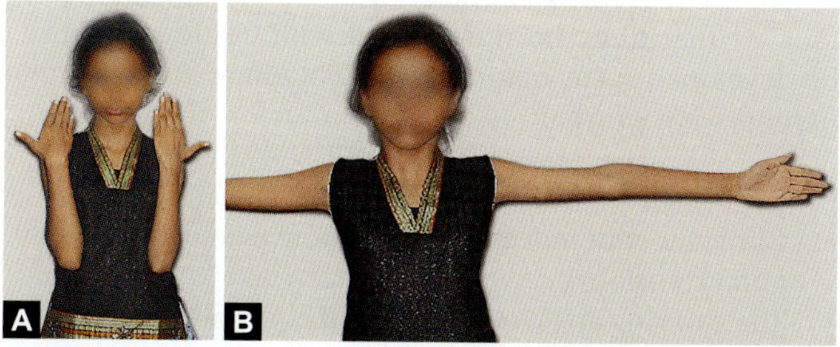

Figs. 11.6A and B: Final clinical results showing full flexion and extension.

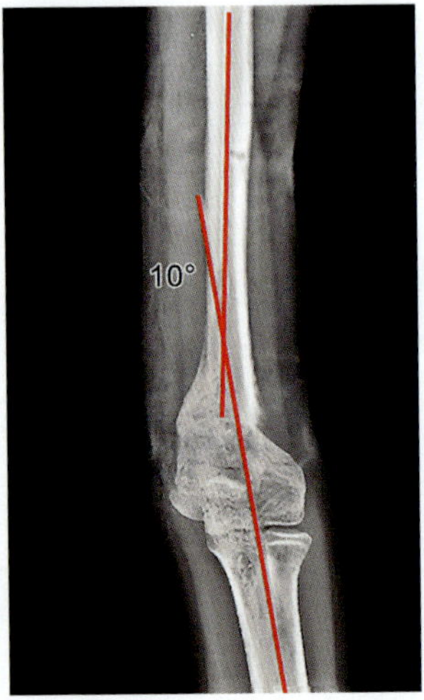

Fig. 11.7: The achievement of normal humerus-elbow-wrist (HEW) angle.

Case 2

Brief Clinical History

A young boy aged six having cubitus varus deformity, right elbow. He had supracondylar fracture at the age of four. At that time, he was treated with casting. However, he developed varus deformity of right elbow for which the parents were worried.

Preoperative Clinical Photos

- Clinically, the movements of elbow were—flexion 140° and extension 5°.
- The carrying angle of the affected elbow was 24° varus.
- The carrying angle of the normal elbow was 6° valgus.
- Clinically the total correction was 30° **(Fig. 11.8)**.

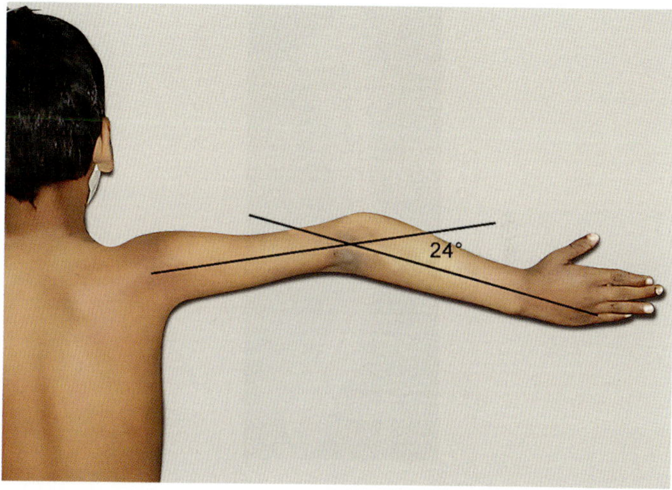

Fig. 11.8: Cubitus varus 24°.

Preoperative Radiographs

- The HEW angle of the affected elbow was 23° varus.
- The HEW angle of the normal elbow was 7° valgus.
- The total correction was 30° **(Figs. 11.9 and 11.10)**.

Treatment Strategies

We planned to apply Ilizarov frame for correction of cubitus varus by supracondylar open wedge osteotomy. Preconstructed frame was prepared with two rings connected with hinges. The angulation of the distal ring was according to the total deformity corrected (30°).

The frame was fixed with the two olive wires and half pins in the distal ring and two olive wires and half pins in the proximal ring. Supracondylar osteotomy was performed just above the olecranon fossa which was confirmed

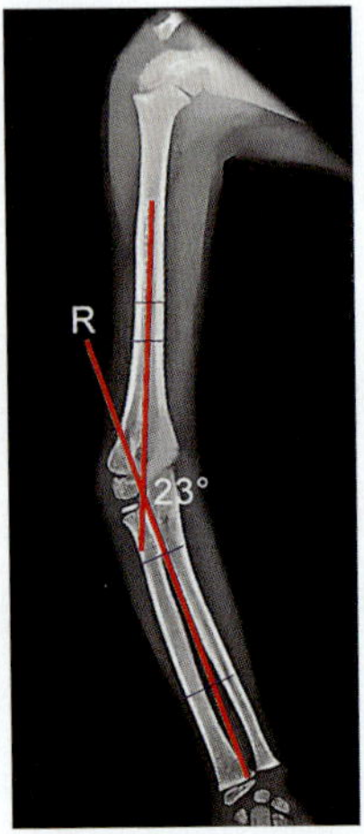

Fig. 11.9: X-ray with 23° varus.

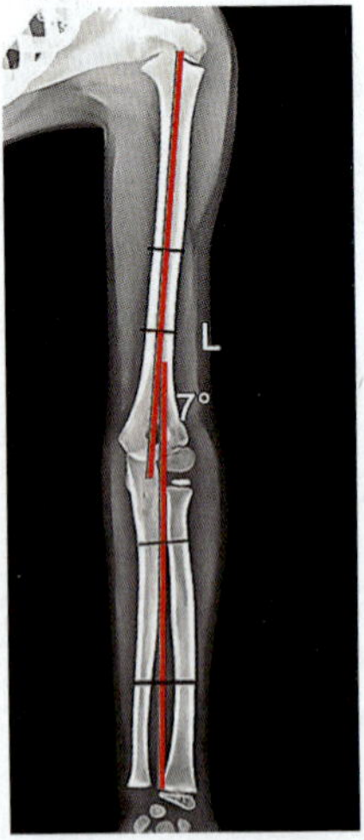

Fig. 11.10: Normal elbow X-ray.

under C-arm. The deformity was corrected by 7th post-operative day. The distraction rate was calculated by the rule of similar triangles. The full correction was achieved and both rings were becoming parallel. The 20° internal rotation was corrected by derotating the distal ring anticlockwise by shifting the threaded rods one hole in clockwise direction, thus the 10° correction was achieved and in the next week further 10° derotation was done by shifting the threaded rods.

Postoperative Management

Proper cleaning of the wires and pins was done. Physiotherapy was started as soon as the pain subsided **(Figs. 11.11 and 11.12)**.

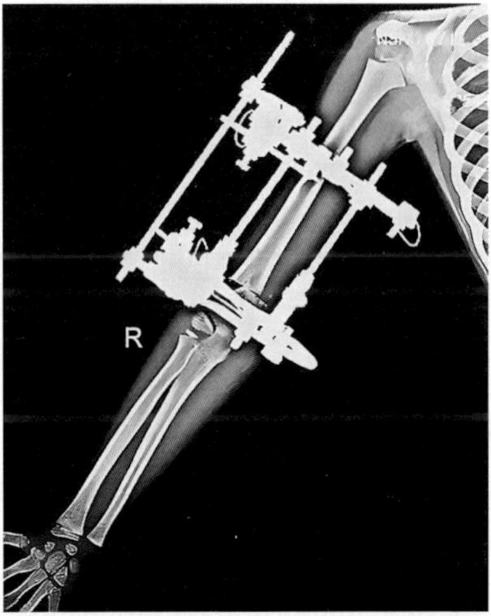

Fig. 11.11: Postoperative X-ray.

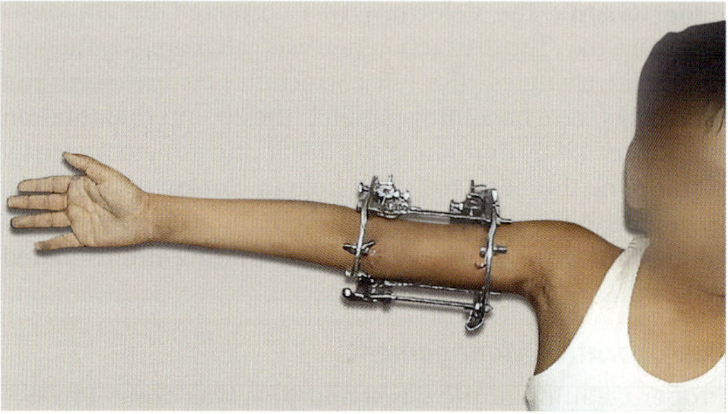

Fig. 11.12: Postoperative clinical photograph.

Removal of the Frame

Frame was removed by eight weeks after confirming the correction clinically and radiologically.

Photographs and Radiographs after Final Correction

At the final follow-up, the deformity was corrected fully and full flexion and extension of elbow were achieved. Radiologically, the final HEW angle was 10° valgus, which was preoperatively 7° **(Figs. 11.13 and 11.14)**.

Case 3

Brief Clinical History

A young boy aged 16 having cubitus varus deformity of right elbow. He had supracondylar fracture at the age of six and was treated by plaster casting. There was a cosmetic deformity at the right elbow and patient was complaining of pain during heavy work.

Preoperative Clinical Photos

- Clinically, the range of movement of elbow was flexion 135° and extension 0°.
- The carrying angle of the affected elbow was 31° varus.

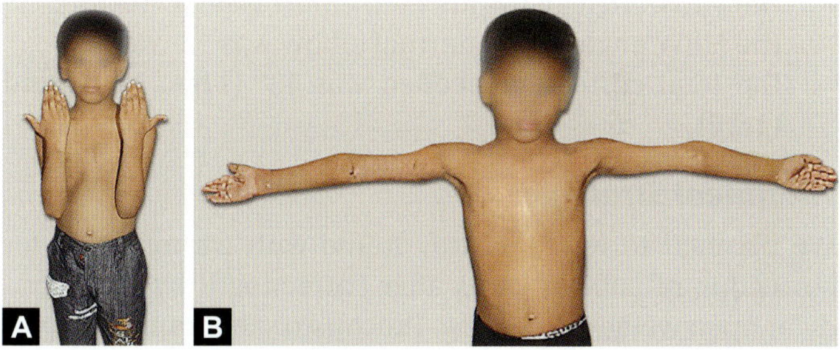

Figs. 11.13A and B: Final photographs.

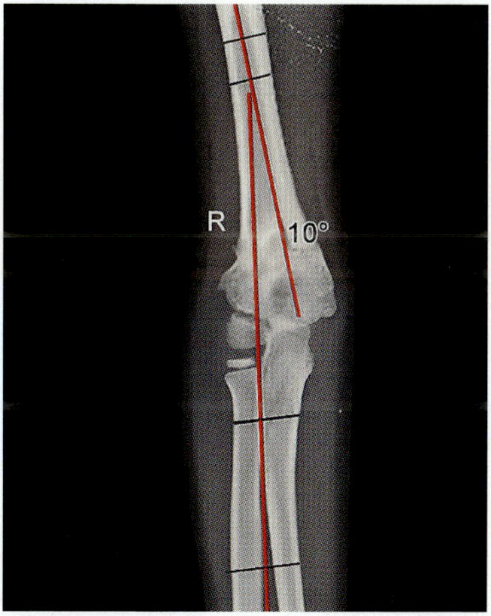

Fig. 11.14: Final X-ray.

- The carrying angle of the normal elbow was 12° valgus.
- Clinically, the total correction needed was 43° **(Fig. 11.15)**.

Preoperative Radiographs

- The HEW angle of the affected elbow was 31° varus.
- The HEW angle of the normal elbow was 12° valgus.
- The total correction needed was 43° **(Figs. 11.16 and 11.17)**.

Treatment Strategies

We planned to apply Ilizarov frame with carbon rings for correction of cubitus varus after correcting it by supracondylar open wedge osteotomy. Preconstructed frame was prepared with two rings connected with juxta-articular hinges.

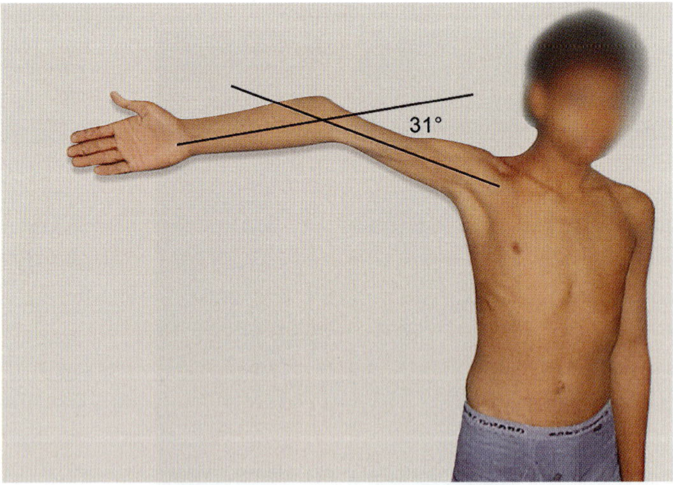

Fig. 11.15: Varus deformity 31°.

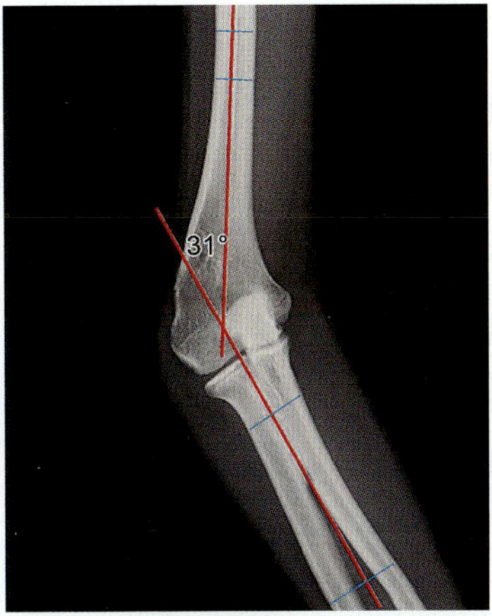

Fig. 11.16: Preoperative X-ray 31° varus.

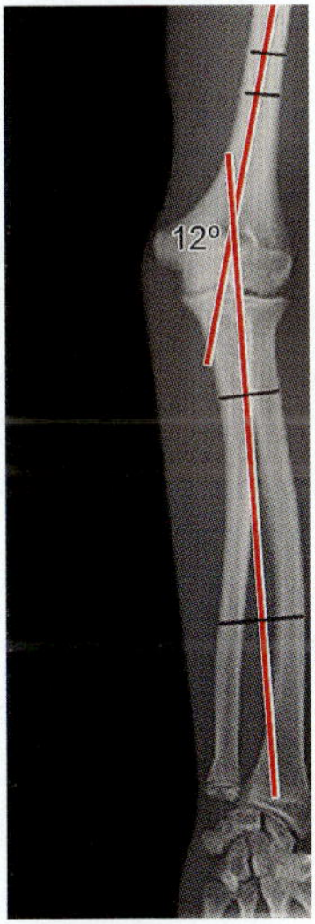

Fig. 11.17: Normal carrying angle.

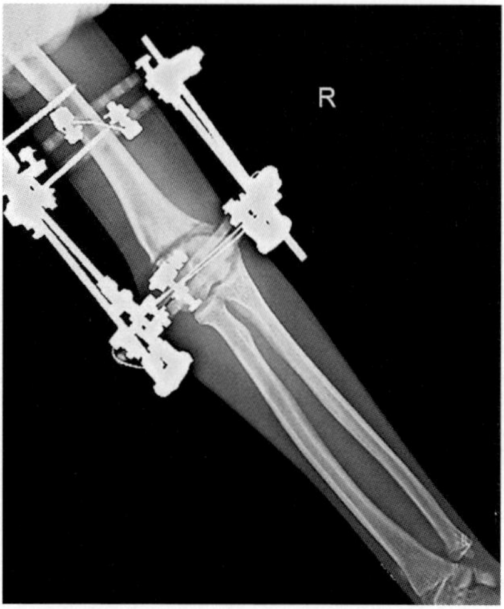

Fig. 11.18: Postoperative X-ray.

The angulation of the distal ring was according to the total corrected deformity (43°) **(Figs. 11.18 and 11.19)**.

The frame was fixed with two olive wires and one half pin in the distal rings and one olive wire and two half pins in the proximal ring. Supracondylar osteotomy was performed just above the olecranon fossa which was confirmed under C-arm. The deformity was corrected after seven days. The distraction rate was calculated by rule of similar triangles. The full correction was achieved and both rings were becoming parallel. The 10° internal rotation was corrected by derotation of the distal ring anticlockwise by shifting the threaded rods one hole in clockwise direction.

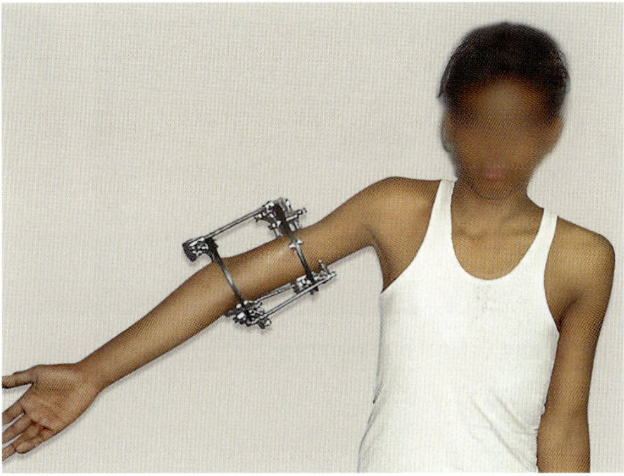

Fig. 11.19: Postoperative photograph.

Postoperative Management

Proper cleaning of the wires and pins was done. Physiotherapy was started as soon as the pain subsided.

Removal of the Frame

Frame was removed after 12 weeks after confirming the correction clinically and radiologically **(Figs. 11.20 and 11.21)**.

Final Clinical Photos and Radiographs

At the final follow-up, cosmetically the deformity was corrected fully and achieved full flexion and extension of elbow. Radiologically, the final HEW angle was 10° valgus, whereas preoperative HEW angle of normal elbow was 7° valgus.

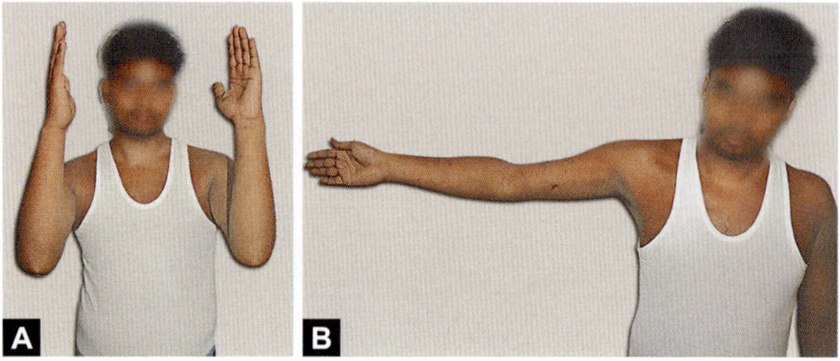

Figs. 11.20A and B: Final photographs.

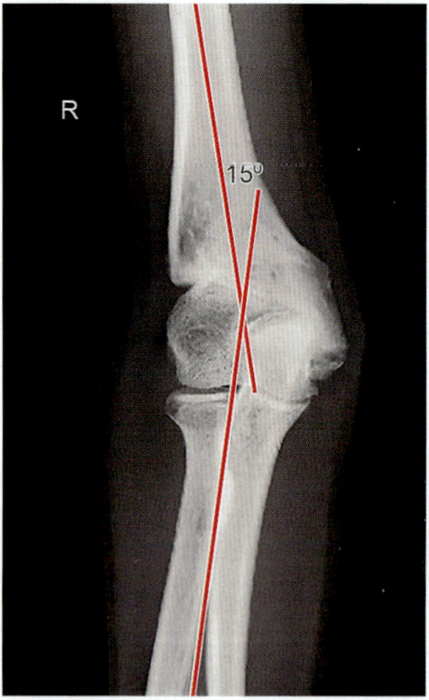

Fig. 11.21: Final X-ray.

Case 4

Brief Clinical History

A young boy aged seven having cubitus varus deformity of left elbow. He had supracondylar fractures at the age of five which was treated with casting. There was a cubitus varus deformity at the right elbow and was complaining of pain during heavy work.

Preoperative Radiographs

- The HEW angle of the affected elbow was 18° varus.
- The HEW angle of the normal elbow was 7° valgus.
- The total correction needed was 25° **(Fig. 11.22)**.

Preoperative Clinical Photos

- Clinically, the range of movements of elbow was flexion 135° and extension 0°.
- The carrying angle of the affected elbow was 19° varus.

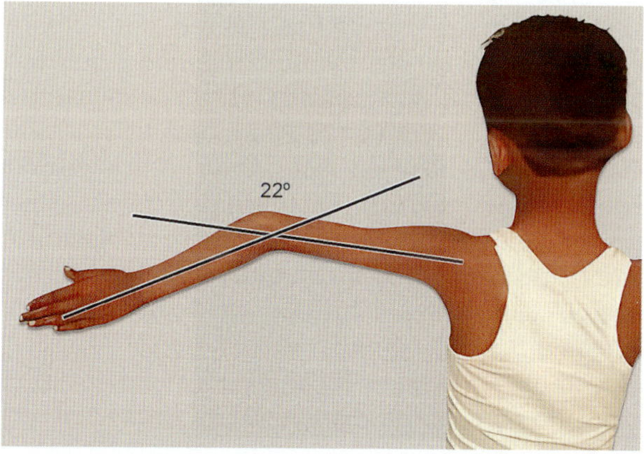

Fig. 11.22: Varus deformity 22°.

- The carrying angle of the normal elbow was 6° valgus.
- Clinically, the total correction needed was 25° **(Figs. 11.23 and 11.24)**.

Treatment Strategies

We planned to apply Ilizarov frame after correction of cubitus varus by supracondylar open wedge osteotomy. Preconstructed frame was prepared with two rings connected with hinges. The angulation of the distal ring was according to the total deformity corrected (25°).

The frame was fixed with the two olive wires in the distal ring and two olive wires and one drop wire in the proximal ring. Supracondylar osteotomy was performed just above the olecranon fossa after confirming under C-arm. The deformity was corrected after postoperative 5th day. The distraction rate was calculated by rule of similar

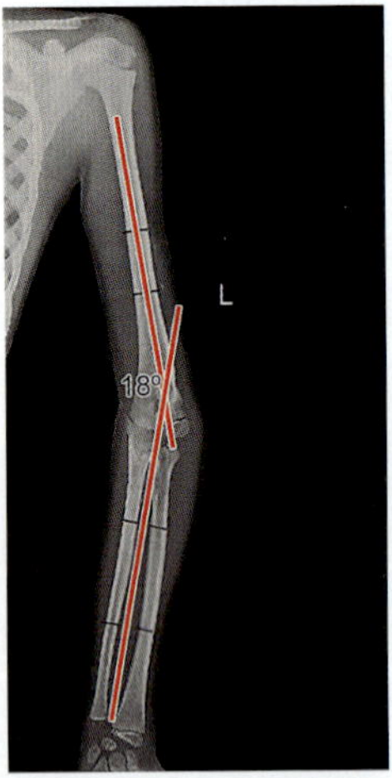

Fig. 11.23: Preoperative X-ray.

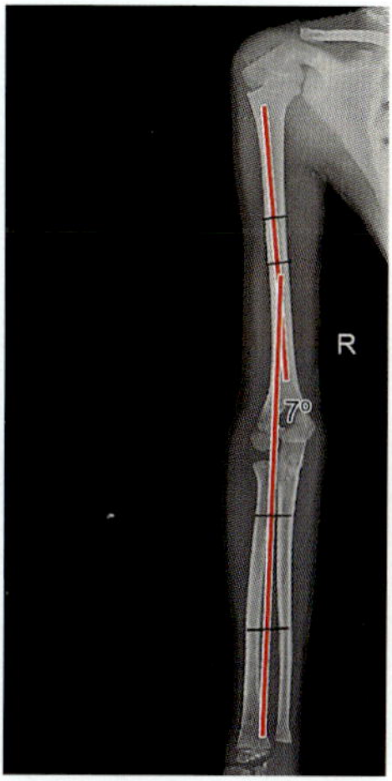

Fig. 11.24: Normal elbow X-ray.

triangles. When the full correction was achieved, both rings became parallel. The 20° internal rotation was corrected by derotation of the distal ring anticlockwise by shifting the threaded rods one hole in clockwise direction, thus the 10° correction was achieved and in the next week, further 10° derotation was done by shifting the threaded rods.

Postoperative Management

Proper cleaning of the wires and pins was done. Physiotherapy was started as soon as the pain subsided **(Figs. 11.25 and 11.26)**.

Removal of the Frame

Frame was removed after 10 weeks after confirming clinically and radiologically.

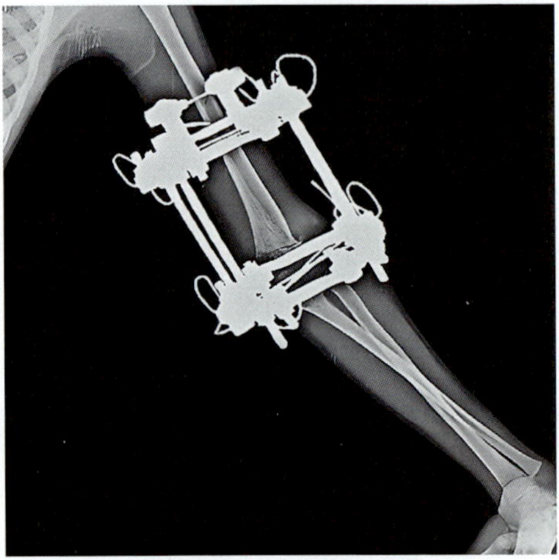

Fig. 11.25: Postoperative X-ray.

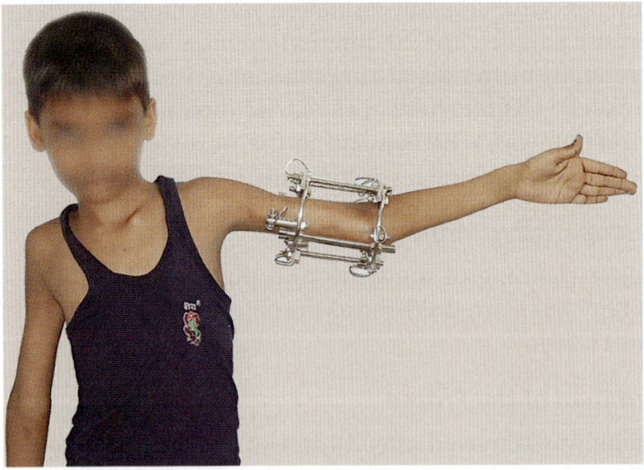

Fig. 11.26: Postoperative clinical photograph.

Final Clinical Photos and Radiographs

At the final follow-up, the deformity was fully corrected with full flexion and extension of elbow. Radiologically, the final HEW angle was 12° valgus which was preoperatively 7° **(Figs. 11.27 and 11.28)**.

Case 5

Brief Clinical History

A young boy aged eight years with cubitus varus deformity of left elbow. He had supracondylar fracture at the age of six years and six months and was treated with plaster casting. There was a cosmetic deformity at the left elbow **(Fig. 11.29)**.

Preoperative Radiographs

- The HEW angle of the affected elbow was 17° varus.
- The HEW angle of the normal elbow was 10° valgus.
- The total correction needed was 27°.

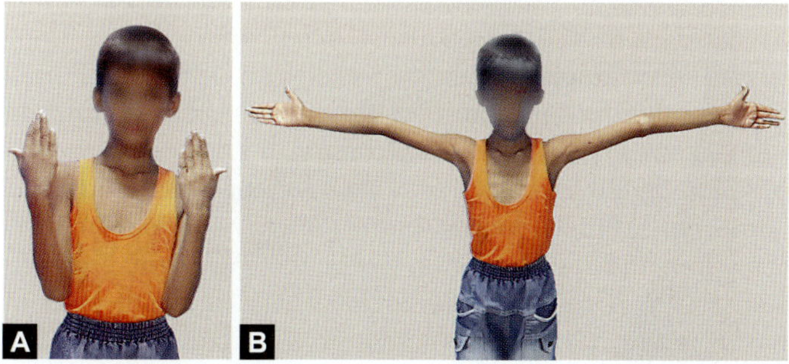

Figs. 11.27A and B: Final clinical photos.

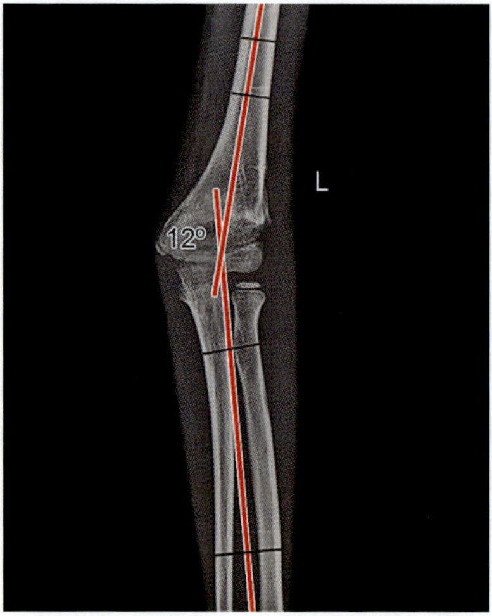

Fig. 11.28: Final X-ray.

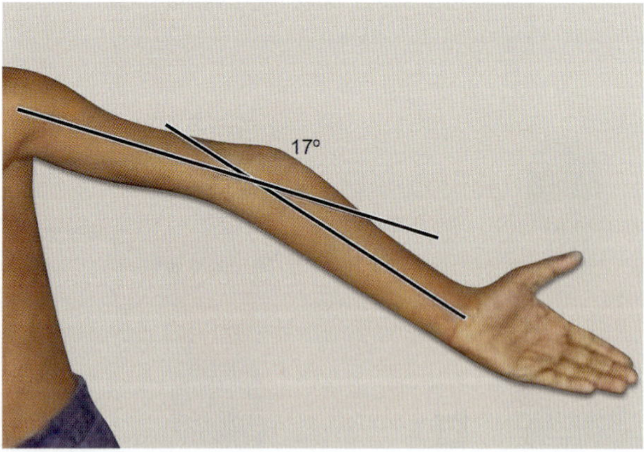

Fig. 11.29: Preoperative photograph.

Preoperative Clinical Photos

- Clinically, the range of movements of elbow was flexion 140° and extension 0°.
- The carrying angle of the affected elbow was 17° varus.
- The carrying angle of the normal elbow was 10° valgus.
- Clinically, the total correction needed was 27° **(Figs. 11.30 and 11.31)**.

Treatment Strategies

We planned to apply Ilizarov frame after correction of cubitus varus by supracondylar open wedge osteotomy. Preconstructed frame was prepared with two rings connected with hinges. The angulation of the distal ring was according to the total deformity corrected (27°).

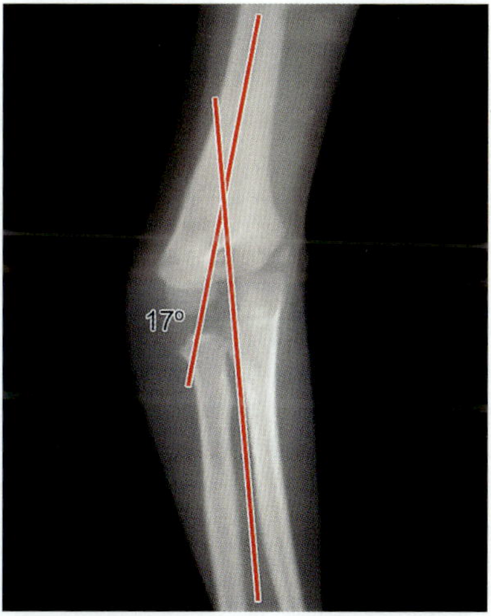

Fig. 11.30: Preoperative X-ray.

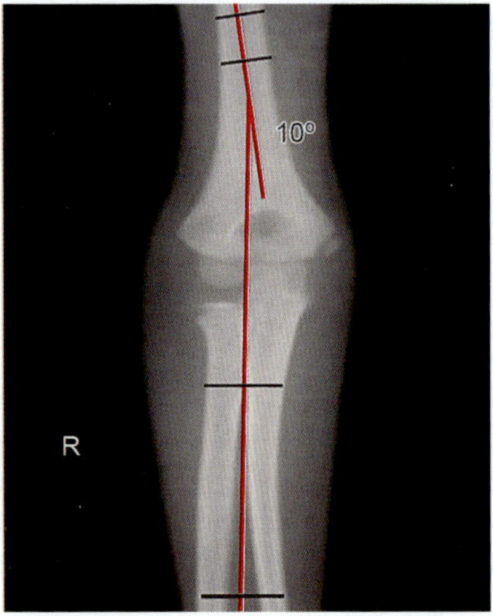

Fig. 11.31: Normal elbow X-ray.

The frame was fixed with the one olive wire and two half pins in the distal rings and two half pins in the proximal ring. Supracondylar osteotomy was performed just above the olecranon fossa and was confirmed under C-arm. The deformity was corrected after postoperative 7th day. The distraction rate was calculated by rule of similar triangles. The full correction was achieved and both rings became parallel. The 20° internal rotation was corrected by derotation of the distal ring anticlockwise by shifting the threaded rods one hole in clockwise direction, thus, the 10° correction was achieved and in the next week, further 10° derotation was done by shifting the threaded rods.

Postoperative Management

Proper cleaning of the wires and pins was done. Physiotherapy was started as soon as the pain subsided **(Figs. 11.32 and 11.33)**.

Removal of the Frame

Frame was removed after nine weeks after confirming the correction clinically and radiologically **(Figs. 11.34 and 11.35)**.

Final Clinical Photos and Radiographs

At the final follow-up, cosmetically the deformity was corrected fully and full flexion and extension of elbow were achieved. Radiologically, the final HEW angle was 10° valgus which was preoperatively 7°.

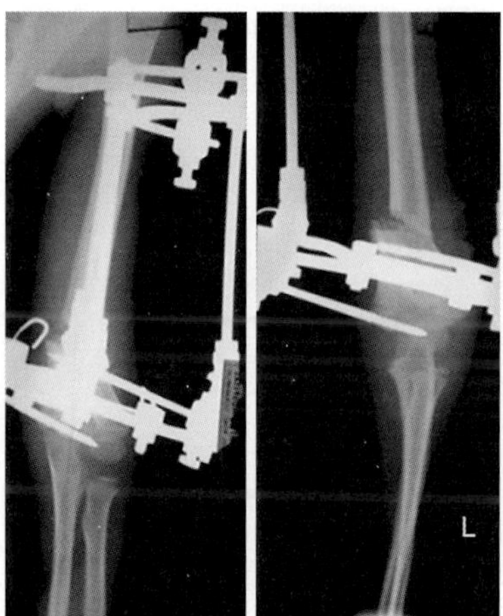

Fig. 11.32: Postoperative X-ray.

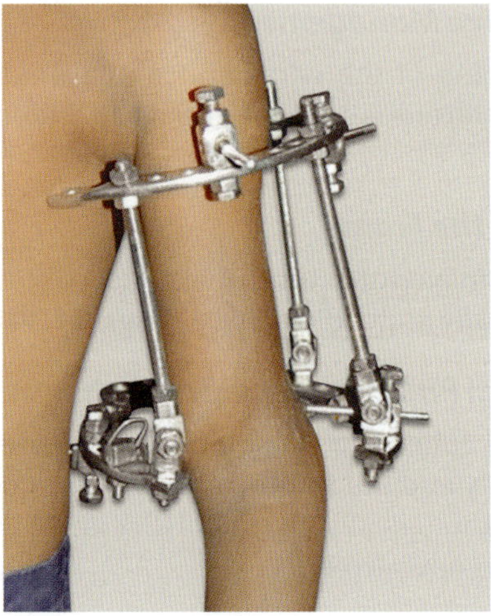

Fig. 11.33: Postoperative photograph.

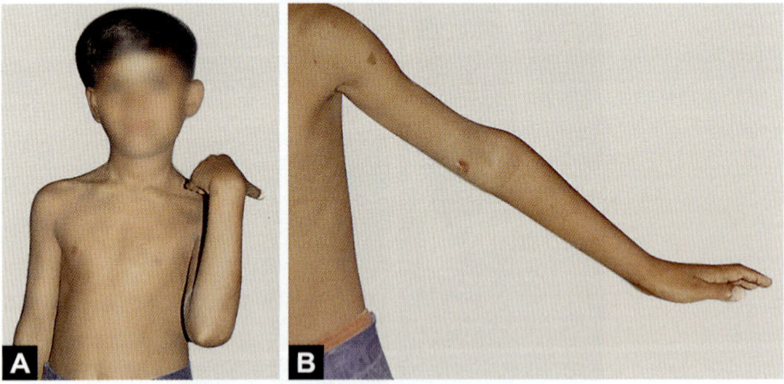

Figs. 11.34A and B: Final clinical photos.

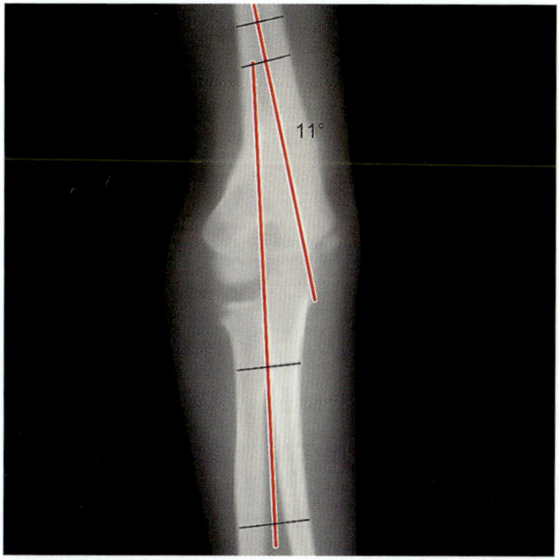

Fig. 11.35: Final X-ray.

CHAPTER

12 Review of Literature

INTRODUCTION

Multiple outcome assessment criteria, or scales, reported in the selected studies included the reports of Oppenheim, modified Oppenheim, Bellemore, Labelle, and Morrey scores; or surgeons' independent scales of outcome based on correction of deformity, range of movement (ROM), alignment, and the presence or absence of complications.

For the purpose of final analysis, complications were classified as "major" or "minor". Major complications were defined as residual varus deformity, nerve injury, infection, loss of fixation leading to reoperation, and growth arrest. Minor complications included loss of fixation or reoperation, unsightly scarring, stiffness, or a prominent lateral condyle.

In patients requiring corrective osteotomy, the mean age was 9.8 years (4–15.7) at the time of correction.

Osteotomy techniques used were:

- Lateral closing wedge ($n = 562$, 62.9%)
- Complex ($n = 182$, 20.4%)
- Dome ($n = 98$, 11.0%)
- Distraction osteogenesis ($n = 37$, 4.1%)
- Medial opening wedge ($n = 15$, 1.7%)

("Complex" osteotomies were defined as those using multiplanar geometry and were described in the literature as step-cut, modified step-cut, translation step-cut, pentalateral, three-dimensional, interlocking wedge, and reverse "V".)

The most common fixation methods used were:

- Kirschner (K) wires/pins (*n* = 424, 46.9%), followed by
- External fixators (*n* = 114, 12.6%),
- Tension bands around screws (*n* = 99, 11.0%)
- Screws alone (*n* = 72, 8.0%)
- Plates (*n* = 37, 4.1%)

Patients in some studies were treated with:
Staples (*n* = 24, 2.7%), a combination of fixation methods or other techniques.

Nerve injury rates in osteotomy series were:

- Complex 2.1% (95% CI 0.1–4.0)
- Dome 4.9% (95% CI 0.0–10.6)
- Lateral wedge 2.7% (95% CI 0.2–5.1)
- Distraction osteogenesis 1.9% (95% CI 0.0–6.6)

Residual varus was the most common complication across all surgical techniques, affecting an estimated 5.9% of patients (95% CI 3.9–7.8).

The overall infection rate was 2.5% (95% CI 1.4–3.5).

Reoperation was needed in less number of patients (2.3%) (95% CI 1.2–3.4).

COMPLICATIONS BY FIXATION METHOD

21.2% of the patients treated with K-wire/pin fixation sustained complications, including residual varus (10.0%), loss of fixation (2.6%), and infection (3.7%).

One-quarter of the patients treated with a tension-band technique sustained complications.

Patients treated with screws alone had 8.7% complications; external fixation (10.0%) had the lowest overall complication rates, although 6.7% of the patients with external fixation have the lowest overall complication rates.

The overall reported nerve injury was 4.2%: 1.9% in lateral approach, 12.1% in medial approach, and 3.7% in posterior approach.

Scarring rate was 1.4% in lateral approach, 8.8% in medial approach, 3.4% in posterior approach.

Bibliography

1. An KN, Morrey BF, Chao EY. Carrying angle of the human elbow joint. J Orthop Res. 1984;1:369-78.
2. Calhoun JH, Li F, Bauford WL, Lehman T, Ledbetter BR, Lowery R. Rigidity of half-pins for the Ilizarov external fixator. Bull Hosp Joint Dis. 1992;52(1):21-6.
3. Chapleau J, Canet F, Petit Y, Laflamme GY, Rouleau DM. Validity of goniometric elbow measurements: Comparative study with a radiographic method. Clin Orthop Relat Res. 2011;469(11):3134-40.
4. Dai L. Radiographic evaluation of Baumann angle in Chinese children and its clinical relevance. J Pediatr Orthop B. 1999;8(3): 197-9.
5. French PR. Varus deformity of the elbow following supracondylar fractures of the humerus in children. Lancet. 1959;2:439-41.
6. Hasegawa M, Suzuki T, Kuroiwa T, Oka Y, Maeda A, Takeda H, et al. Reliability and validity of measurement of the Humerus-Elbow-Wrist angle in children. JB JS Open Access. 2017;2(1):e0012.
7. Herzenberg JE, Waanders NA. Calculating rate and duration of distraction for deformity correction with the Ilizarov technique. Orthop Clin North Am. 1991;22:601-11.
8. Horstmann HM, Blyakher AA, Quartararo LG, Cavalier R. Treatment of cubitus varus with osteotomy and Ilizarov external fixation. Am J Orthop. 2000;29:389-91.
9. Karatosun V, Alekberov C, Alici E, Ardicx CO, Aksu G. Treatment of cubitus varus using the Ilizarov technique of distraction osteogenesis. J Bone Joint Surg Br. 2000;82(7):1030-3.
10. Ozkan C, Dogramacı Y, Kalacı A, Güls¸ en M, Bayram H. Results of using Ilizarov distraction osteogenesis technique for the treatment of cubitus varus deformities in adults. Arch Orthop Trauma Surg. 2010;130(4):489-95.
11. Paley D. Osteotomy concepts and frontal plane realignment. In: Paley D (Ed). Principles of Deformity Correction, 1st edition. Berlin: Springer-Verlag; 2002. pp. 99-154.

12. Piskin A, Tomak Y, Sen C, Tomak L. The management of cubitus varus and valgus using Ilizarov method. J Bone Joint Surg Br. 2007;89(12):1615-9.
13. Podolsky A, Chao EY. Mechanical performance of Ilizarov circular external fixators in comparison with other external fixators. Clin Orthop Relat Res. 1993;(293):61-70.
14. Sangwan MM, Marya KM, Siwach RC, Singh Z, Devgan A. Cubitus varus correction by distraction osteogenesis. Indian J Med Sci. 2002;56(4):165-71.
15. Smith L. Deformity following supracondylar fractures of the humerus. J Bone Joint Surg Am. 1960;42(2):235-52.
16. Song HR, Cho SM, Seoug ST, Park YJ, Koo KH. Supracondylar osteotomy with Ilizarov fixation for elbow deformity in adults. J Bone Joint Surg Br. 1997;19(B):748-52.
17. Yamamoto I, Ishii S, Usui M, Ogino T, Kaneda K. Cubitus varus deformity following supracondylar fracture of the humerus. A method of measuring rotational deformity. Clin Orthop Relat Res. 1985;201:179-85.

Index

Page numbers followed by *f* refer to figure.

D

E

F

G

H

I

J

K

L

M

N

O